THE HEARING TRANSFORMATION

THE FACTS YOU NEED TO KNOW

to change your **life**, improve **relationships**, maintain your **independence**, and improve **cognitive function**

DR. MELINDA 'SUNNI' MCBRIDE, AUD
DR. KEITH N. DARROW, PHD

EIA MEDIA GROUP

The Hearing Transformation: The facts you need to know to change your life, improve relationships, maintain your independence, and improve cognitive function — by Dr. Melinda 'Sunni' McBride, AuD, and Dr. Keith N. Darrow, PhD

Project Director: Jared M. Brader, MBA
Editor: Kelly Martin
Associate Editor: Kristin Lewis
Graphics: Steve Ruesch
Cover & Interior Design: Five J's Design, FiveJsDesign.com

First Printing: December 2018

ISBN: 978-1-7314-1279-9

Dr. McBride's Acknowledgements

To my father, the first "Dr. McBride," a family practice doctor for over 40 years. Thank you for sharing your love of medicine and patients with me. Thank you for suggesting I look into majoring in Audiology.

I am also grateful to my husband, Jim Gerszewski, for working by my side since 2007. It has been a fun ride! There have been many late nights spent at the office. And who knew that you could see the world talking about hearing? Europe, South America, Mexico and China have been on the travel list, to mention a few stops along the way.

Thanks to my kids who put up with a mother going back to college to get her doctoral degree when she was in her 40's.

I have an amazing team at South Bay Hearing & Mission Audiology. You were handpicked, one by one. It is the special sprit that you exude to our patients which makes them keep coming back and sending their friends. You can't bottle or prescribe enthusiasm and true caring. But our patients feel it.

The hearing care management team, Audigy, was instrumental in helping me develop business systems to make us more efficient. You have pushed us to achieve goals that were inconceivable when we began this journey.

And thanks to AudExperts and AUDMA for showing us how to transform again, to utilize digital tools and Big Data to help us reach more people who need our help.

TABLE OF CONTENTS

THE HEARING TRANSFORMATION

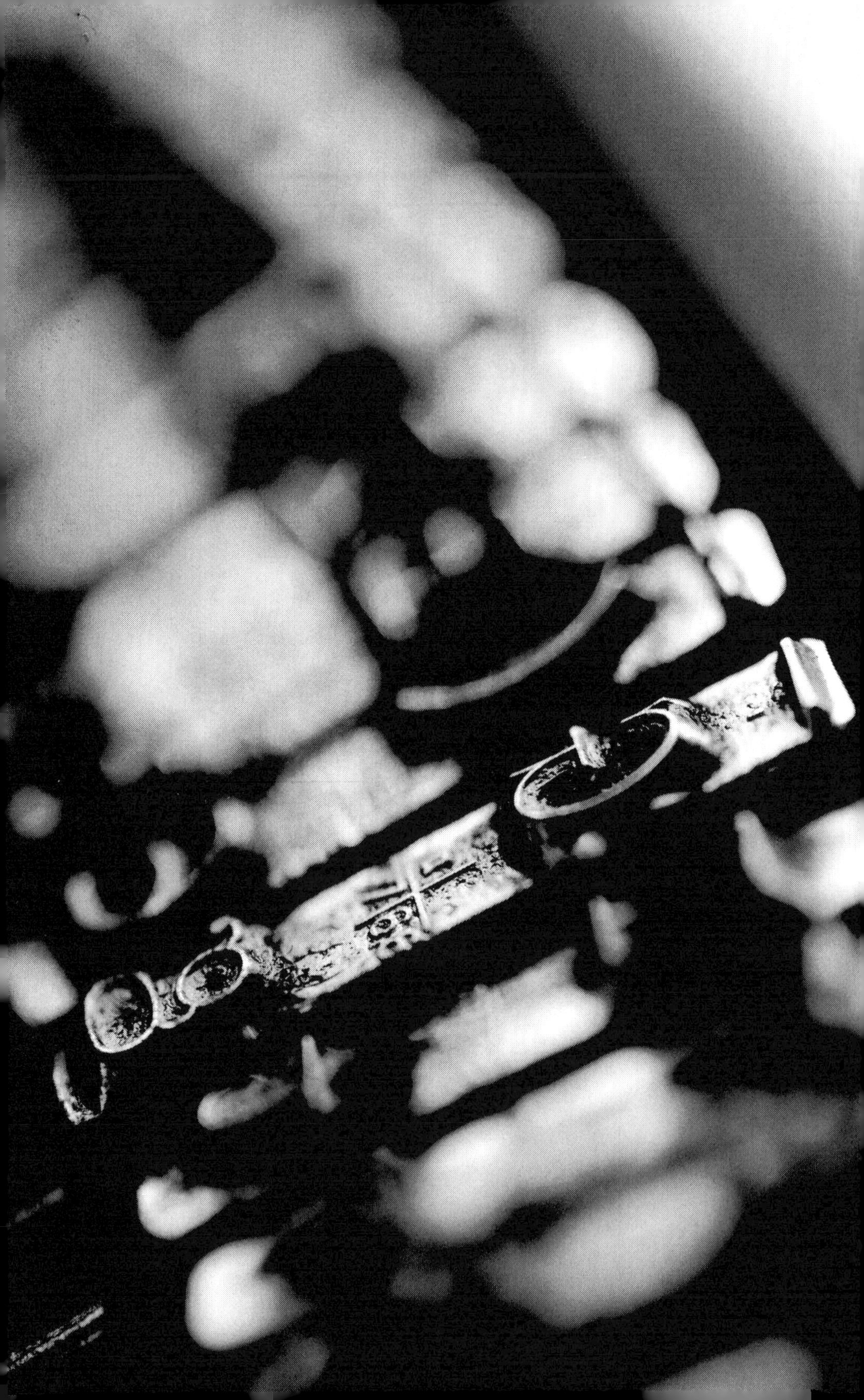

ABOUT THE AUTHORS

DR. SUNNI MCBRIDE, AUD,

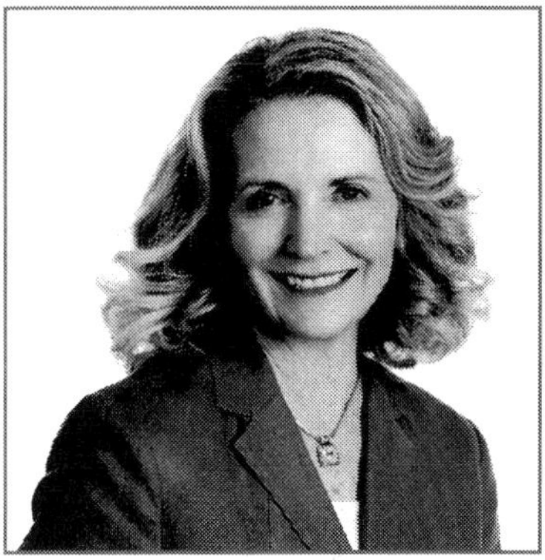

founder of South Bay Hearing, is leading the movement to medically treat hearing loss and the associated cognitive deprivation in Los Angeles. By working alongside her team of doctors, including neuroscientist Dr. Keith Darrow, NeuroTechnology™ Treatment Specialists, and her entire patient experience team, Dr. McBride and her team are able to focus on medically treating your hearing loss, tinnitus, and the associated cognitive impacts.

Dr. McBride is described as an 'Innovative Audiology Leader' by Dr. Keith Darrow, her co-author on this Amazon #1 best-selling, patient-focused book, *The Hearing Transformation.* When in the care of Dr. McBride and her team, your treatment will be based upon YOUR background, situation, and experience and will follow proven protocols known to restore hearing clarity and reduce the risk of cognitive decline and Dementia.

Her impact on our organization, the profession, and the world includes:

- being trained by Dr. Keith Darrow, the only Harvard and M.I.T. trained neuroscientist and audiologist in the world, as part of the Excellence in Audiology Movement which focuses your hearing loss treatment on sound medical and neuroscience technology rather than traditional hearing aids;
- restoring hearing clarity for thousands of individuals in Southern California with hearing loss just like yours;
- being voted South Bay's Best Audiologist every year since 2008;

- being the only AudigyCertified™ Practice in the community since 2011;
- being the first Lyric™ Treatment Provider in Southern California;
- lecturing and coaching private audiology practices in countries around the world;
- being featured on CBS and cable television channels;
- serving as an adjunct professor at California State Los Angeles University;
- her team treating over 1,000 patients in Guadalajara, Mexico, and over 3,500 patients in China as part of her philanthropic activities;
- and co-sponsoring the Senior Aging Expo.

DR. KEITH N. DARROW

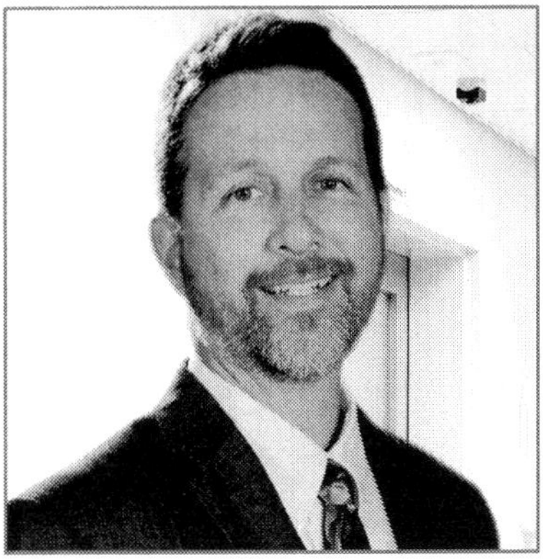

is an expert in Speech and Hearing Bioscience and Technology with a doctoral degree from the joint Massachusetts Institute of Technology (M.I.T) and Harvard Medical School program. He is a former Clinical Professor at Northeastern University (Boston, MA) and is currently a tenured professor at Worcester State University.

Dr. Darrow's clinical experience is vast and includes a clinical fellowship at the Department of Otolaryngology at Brigham and Women's Hospital (Boston, MA) and a trainingship at the Audiology Department in the East Orange (NJ) Veterans Association Hospital. He is the owner of the Hearing and Balance Centers of New England and founder of the Healthy Hearing Foundation of New England, as well as a board member of the Sound of Life Foundation (both non-profit organizations dedicated to providing education and hearing health care for those in need). He was recently named the Director of Audiology Research at Intermountain Audiology and has chosen to lead the Excellence In Audiology movement across the country.

Dr. Darrow is a nationally recognized speaker, trainer, and researcher and has been conducting research at the Massachusetts Eye and Ear Infirmary for over fifteen years. His publications and research have been cited over 550 times. On a personal note, Dr. Darrow and his wife Laura have three children (Ella, Mae and Charlie) who love to ski and travel to National Parks together. He also serves on the board of directors for the Worcester County Reserve Deputy Sheriffs Association and provides countless hours of volunteer service in his communities.

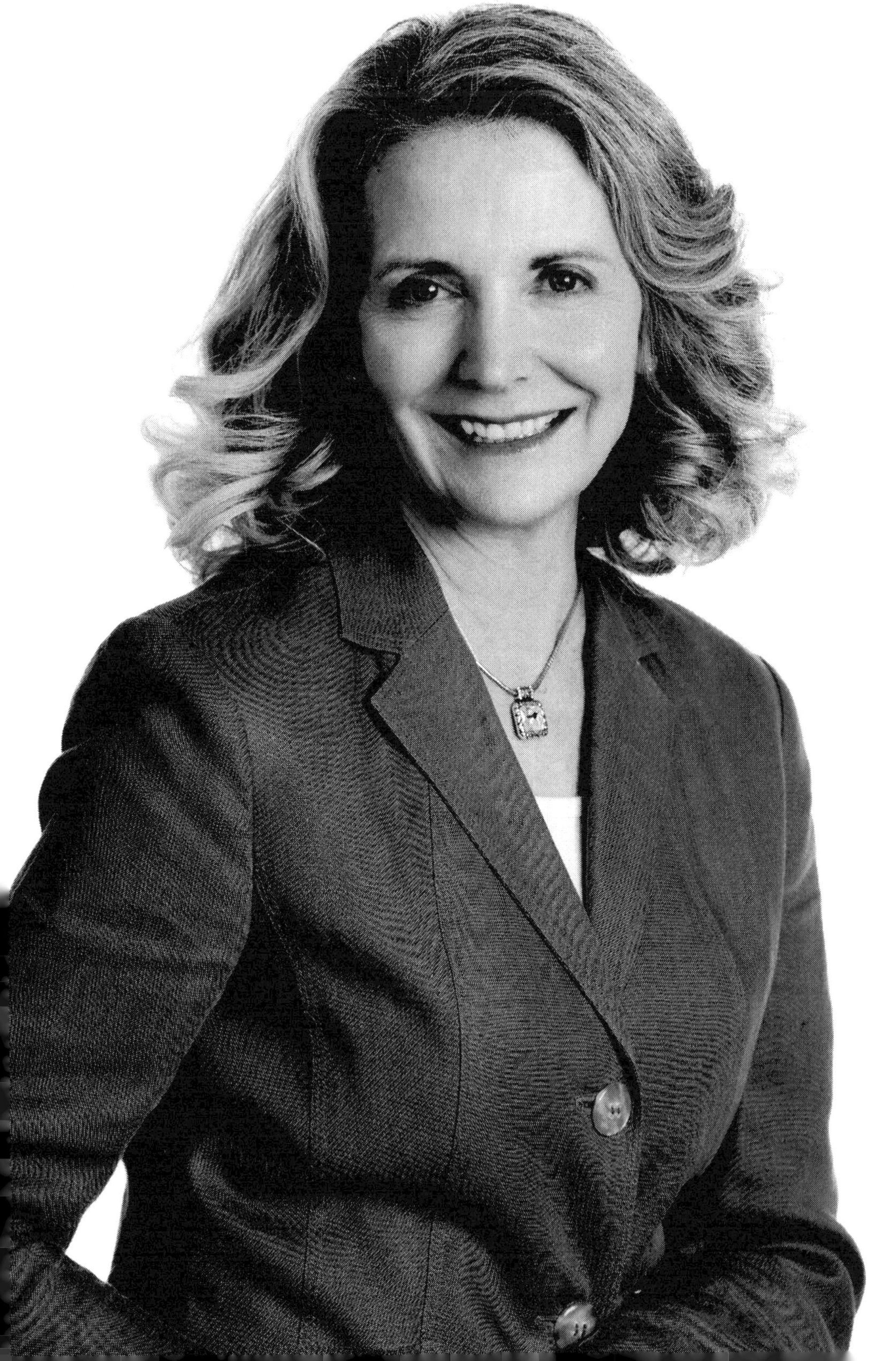

INTERVIEW
WITH DR. MCBRIDE

SPEAKERS

John Melley (**JM**) | Dr. Sunni McBride (**DSM**) | Participants (**P**)

Audio 1

[This is On the Air with John Melley, a compelling interview program featuring today's innovative business leaders. Join us as we explore the creative solutions and unique products and services being developed for today's consumers and how businesses are thriving in today's complex marketplace. Now here's your host John Melley.]

JM: Hello and welcome to the program. Do you or a loved one have impaired hearing? Did you know that hearing problems can lead to social isolation and increase your risk for other health problems? You want to remain independent and live an active life as you age. Well, all of these can be affected by the quality of your hearing. If you or someone you care for has impaired hearing, this is a program you will want to pay attention to.

My guest today is Dr. Sunni McBride and she's here to talk about hearing loss and what you can do about it to maintain a high quality of life. Before we dive in, let me tell you a little bit about my guest today. Dr. McBride received her Doctorate from the University of Florida and she started her practice in 2007. She is one of the top Lyric hearing aid providers in the United States. She's the co-sponsor of The Senior Aging Expo.

She has provided thousands of hearing aids to needy people on mission trips to Mexico and China. She has been featured on CBS's "This is LA." She taught audiology classes at California State Los Angeles University and she promotes and presents hearing and prevention awareness to local and national organizations. When she's not in the office, if you can believe this, she might be playing with her 26 grandchildren, skiing with family or enjoying the ocean and the mountains. But she also says you shouldn't be surprised if you drive by their office late at night and still see the lights on. Dr. McBride, thank you for being on the show today. I could go on with all of your accomplishments but we need to get started. How are you?

DSM: Thank you John. That was very kind of you. Doing well today, thank you.

JM: Very good. Well, it's very kind of you to take time to be with us today and talk about this important topic. Before we start talking about the importance of treating hearing loss, I was wondering if you could tell everyone how you got started on the road to becoming a Doctor of Audiology.

DSM: Sure. Well, I was really fortunate. My father was a family practice physician and he wanted to keep his teenage daughter out of trouble. So he invited me to come and work in his office after school. So for many years in high school and college, I had the opportunity to work by my father's side. He was one of those old-fashioned family practice doctors that really took time and actually talked to their patients. His patients just loved him. I learned so much from him about patient care, compassion and really being kind to people.

So when I went off to college, of course I wanted to be like my dad and I was going to go into medical school. But then I met a really cute fellow and decided that what I really wanted to do was get married and raise a family. So I managed to get my Master's of Communication Disorders by the time we both left college. I actually got to work part-time as an audiologist until my number two child was born.

I took time off from work. I spent 20 years at home and raised a family of five children, which was exactly what I really wanted to do with my life. It was a wonderful time to be home with my kids. And then they started to go to college, which was – what do you know- EXPENSIVE! And so I thought, I've got a brain. I've got a degree. Let's see if I can help out a little bit here in the family.

So I actually called the gentleman I had worked for 20 years previously and he said, "Come back and work for me." I said, "Really? I don't remember much." He said, "That's OK. I will teach you everything you need to know."

So I went back first part-time. Audiology had changed. When I first went to college, we didn't do anything with hearing aids. But by then, hearing aids have become a focus of the industry and the business. I was quickly acquiring new skills. And then, at that time, across the country, colleges were starting to offer a new degree, a Doctor of Audiology degree. Instead of doing a PhD that was research-based, the Doctor of Audiology degree was clinically-based.

JM: OK.

DSM: These were first offered as long-distance programs. So I did mine through the University of Florida. We met here at the House Ear Institute every two months for two years and I was able to get my Doctor of Audiology degree in California in about 2000. I think I was one of the first Doctors of Audiology degree granted in California because I jumped on it as soon as it was available. I really wanted to bring my knowledge and skills to the current level available. The degree has served me well in the years since.

JM: Obviously you come from a medical family background. What was it about audiology specifically that attracted you?

DSM: It was really presented to me as an alternative to full practice medicine and something that I could do part-time as a woman. When I actually began to work with the patients, oh, what a joy it was.

When I grew up, I had two sets of very loving grandparents. So for me to be helping people about their age was easy. Both of my grandfathers had significant hearing loss. I knew what it was like to sit around the table and watch my grandfather kind of fade into Lala Land because he couldn't hear what was going on. My other grandfather, he turned his hearing aid up, so he could hear the conversation. Then it would start whistling and grandma would say, "You're whistling pop. Turn your hearing aid down."

So he would dutifully turn it down. But then he couldn't hear and after a while, he tried to turn it up just a little bit and eeh-eeh-eeh, "You're whistling pop!" So I saw what these men suffered through. We didn't really have deep relationships because we really couldn't communicate. Now to be able to work with people and to be able to change their lives and give them the joy of hearing back again, it was more moving than I ever thought it would be. And I didn't have to hurt people or do surgery. So that was pretty good.

JM: Well, that sounds fascinating. My dad wears hearing aids. So I can – yeah, I can understand what you just described with your grandfather. So it's an interesting thing. I want to talk to you about the impact that hearing loss has on the family but I need to take a quick break…

Audio 2

JM: Welcome back. My guest today is Dr. Sunni McBride and we were talking about hearing loss and her journey in becoming a Doctor of Audiology. Doctor, just before the break, we were talking about your grandfathers and how they had hearing loss and how it was difficult for them to participate in the conversations.

You mentioned something that was kind of sad to me: you didn't have deep relationships with them because they weren't able to really communicate on a total level, just because they couldn't hear all of the conversation around them.

I wanted to talk to you about the impact of hearing loss on not just the person who has it but in their family and their friends and those that are close to them.

DSM: Yes, it's really sad. There's a statement that says when one person in the family has hearing loss, actually the whole family has hearing loss because they all have to learn how to deal with it. I had a family come in and said, "You know, my dad started answering questions wrong. It was so funny. We started to keep a journal about it because he just would give the funniest responses. Now it's not funny anymore."

JM: Yeah.

DSM: He had been living with it for so long and it had gotten so overwhelming. Sometimes I see a stubborn person with hearing loss. They say, "Well, if my wife would just speak up, I would be fine." They don't realize that someone will speak up for about 20 seconds.Then we all sink back into our comfort level of speech. It's just normal and natural and it's hard to be forced and raise your voice all the time.

I see so many people who are so frustrated. The wife will come in and she's ready to kill him because she thinks, "He doesn't care about me anymore. He doesn't pay attention to me. He doesn't want to talk to me." But actually, he just can't hear her. So it's just easier for him not to carry on a conversation. It doesn't really have all those other emotional overtones. But it picks up those emotional overtones over time. So I say that we do a lot of marriage counseling. The husband would say, "Well, if she would just speak more clearly, I would be fine." I say, "Guess what. She speaks standard American English just fine."

JM: You just can't hear it.

DSM: Yes. You're just not hearing it. One of the things about hearing loss is that it creeps up on us usually slowly. So most people say, "Well, I can hear. I hear the pots and pans. I hear this. I can hear that."

But what they missed are the specific frequencies that provide the clarity of speech. So in English, there are lots of ambiguous words. If you don't hear the word "pat" with a T on the end, it could be the word "pass" with an S on the end or with a T-H on the end and it completely changes the meaning of the word.

Those little sounds are the high frequency sounds that are the first to go. If you're looking at someone, you're kind of reading their lips even though you don't realize you are and your brain is kind of figuring it out from the context of the sentence. You can figure it out for a while. So people get by. But there's a cost to doing all that mentally and we can get into that.

But over time, it becomes a situation so that anytime a person turns away and starts talking, people say, "They should be looking at me." Well, that's because it's louder and you're reading their lips. Those are all things that help people with hearing loss. But yes, when someone in the family has hearing challenges, it's a challenge for everyone.

JM: That's interesting and it's – you're talking to me. I'm sitting here. I'm a radio guy and so I've spent a lot of time in rooms with headphones on and speakers that have probably been too loud and I'm kind of chuckling because you're saying things that I know my wife is dealing with, with me. But I'm only 51. So …

DSM: Yes.

JM: … I could be too young for this stuff, right?

DSM: I get a lot of responses like that from people that are your age, but what people don't realize is that hearing loss can occur at any age. Fifty percent of the people with significant hearing loss in this country are under the age of 60.

JM: Wow.

DSM: And 50 percent are over the age of 60. Well, that becomes compressed in that upper age group. It's more concentrated and so we think, well, hearing loss occurs in old people, which it does. But there are plenty of younger people with hearing challenges. Hearing loss is the number one birth defect and thanks to the good work of some audiologists, we now have national screening of babies in hospitals. They can actually test babies to find out if they're totally deaf or not. That helps them get on the road to early therapy and assistance. So we have much better care for hearing-impaired children these days.

But it's not uncommon for people who have had noise exposure, who have been in the military, who have been to loud concerts or maybe who just have bad genes to have started with hearing loss sooner. I asked one gentleman, "Were you exposed to loud noises growing up?" He said, "Well, I grew up in the '60s, in the age of sex, drugs and rock and roll."

JM: Yeah.

DSM: And I said, "Well, you obviously had more fun than I did."

JM: Oh, man. Yeah, well –

DSM: So lots of things can contribute to hearing loss.

JM: Yeah.

DSM: It's all cumulative, you know. I mean shooting guns in a shooting range, even if you wear hearing protection can cause damage. In a shooting range, that enclosed space keeps all that volume in there. The sound waves get transmitted through your skull and still get into the ear, even though you're wearing ear plugs and ear muffs.

So intense sounds can only be muffled so much and it's all cumulative. People say, "Oh, I went to concerts years ago." Well, guess what. It's kind of like sunburn. Guess what. It all adds up.

JM: Really? Wow. How does that happen? I mean you hear the sound once. Is it just literally wear and tear on the hardware?

DSM: Yes, that's interesting. Of course it all depends on the intensity, the loudness and the duration, the time exposed of the sound. So the louder the sound, the less time it takes to damage the ears. Encased in the skull is the inner ear. We call it the cochlea. It literally looks like a little snail shell.

JM: Right.

DSM: It's the most fascinating structure in the body. It's really like a hose within a hose. It's filled with fluid, lined with little tiny hair cells and when the sound vibrations get transmitted down that fluid, the little hair cells vibrate. It's just like seaweed in the ocean. If you've been in the ocean and a wave comes along, the seaweed vibrates. Well, that's what's going on in your inner ear.

JM: Wow.

DSM: Only each one of those hair cells is tied to a nerve that goes up to the brain. So when that hair cell wiggles, it fires a nerve impulse, so that you can get a message up to the brain.

When you have a loud sound, those really strong vibrations slam into the cochlea and start to destroy hair cells. The body is very redundant. We've got lots of hair cells and so a person might damage a few. Maybe you don't really know there's hearing loss. Then you do it some more and it damages a few more.

Have you ever been to a concert or something where maybe your ears ring a little bit and you're hearing sounds a little muffled?

JM: Yeah.

DSM: And then the next morning, you get up and it has all gone away.

JM: Yeah, yeah. I've been there.

DSM: Well, that's what we call a temporary threshold shift. You actually damaged some of your hearing and then it came back. When you do that time after time, it's like going down a step but not coming all the way back and going down another step and not coming all the way back. So it's just a gradual progression. And over time, the nerves that no longer are connected to the hair cells die off.

JM: Wow. OK. So it's real.

DSM: Yes!

JM: Not all just in my head, is it?

DSM: No, and hard to ignore.

JM: Well, that's true. I'm looking at the clock. We need to take a quick break. But when we come back, let's talk some more about this and what do you say to some of these, "Oh, I'm too young for that" stuff. OK?

DSM: OK.

JM: All right. We will be right back after this.

Audio 3

JM: Welcome back. My guest today is Dr. Sunni McBride and we're discussing hearing loss and how important it is to take care of your hearing. You may be dealing with a hearing loss even if you're not aware of it.

Before the break, we were talking about – I've told you. I'm a radio guy. I've been to a fair share of loud rock concerts. I play the drums and other things and I'm catching myself or catching my wife repeating and all of that. But like I said before, I'm just 51. I feel like I'm kind of – hearing aids are for older folks. I'm too young for that. What do you say?

DSM: Well, I understand the feeling. For example, I put off wearing glasses until my late 40s when I absolutely had to do something about it. So I understand the feeling that people don't want to have more hardware or anything else to deal with for as long as possible.

A few things that you need to consider. First off, you're at work and you're asking people to repeat what they say all the time or you're kind of leaning in with one ear, maybe trying to do it cautiously, so nobody notices. But guess what. Everybody does notice. People around you know you have hearing loss. I have a daughter who worked for a national company and her regional rep had hearing loss. She said, "Mom, it's almost embarrassing. Everybody knows he has hearing loss. But he won't do anything about it."

Studies actually show that untreated hearing loss can cause decreased income. So who wants that? We don't want that! Then you have to understand that the ear really is connected to the brain. The ear's job is to pick up sound waves and to change them into nerve impulses that go up to the brain. All of our listening and understanding occur in the brain in the auditory cortex. It's on each side of your brain.

When you are missing half of the information in the cochlea, you're missing half of the stimulation in that part of the brain. Guess what happens. You're an exercise person. What happens when you don't stimulate things?

JM: You use it or lose it, right?

DSM: That's right.

JM: yeah.

DSM: And the brain actually begins to change and to shrink. Now they've done MRIs where you can compare a normal brain to a brain with untreated hearing loss and it's pretty easy to see the differences that untreated hearing loss can cause over time.

So every time you think, "Well, I'm getting by. I'm doing OK. I don't want to look old. I will just fake it until I make it," type of thing, there are changes going on in your brain. I tell people it's kind of like having a wilted flower. Have you ever given your wife some flowers? She let them wilt. You add a little water to the plant and they perk back up again.

JM: Yeah.

DSM: Because the brain is so plastic, if we catch it early on, we can reorganize the brain. If you wait too long, you go to water that wilted flower, you've been away on vacation, guess what. It's too late and it's not going to respond as well. You can't just look at a hearing test and really understand how the brain is going to respond to normal hearing again.

When I was a kid at school, we were taught that we were born with a certain number of brain cells and all they did was die throughout our life.

JM: Yeah.

DSM: But now we know that that's really not true, that the brain does regenerate and the brain does develop new nerve pathways. That's why they're telling you to learn Chinese and to take up music at an older age because you're doing new and different things and you're expanding your brain. Well, the same is true with giving hearing back through hearing aids. As you re-stimulate the parts of your brain, you're trying to reorganize it and develop new neural pathways, which will help to stave off cognitive decline, which is something we all want to forestall.

JM: I have a question I want to ask you. You've heard the argument probably. You get your eyes checked and they say, "You need to wear glasses," and you start to wear the glasses and your eyesight just gets used to having the glasses and your eyes get weaker.

So then you're going to need a stronger prescription down the road. First of all, is that accurate? If it is, does the same thing happen with hearing aids? Is the hearing aid just going to degrade hearing over time?

DSM: Good question. I'm not an eye specialist. But it's my understanding that the focus of the eye is maintained by muscles and muscle control of the eyes. So I suppose you could make the argument that if your eye doesn't have to work so hard because now you're wearing glasses, that maybe the muscles aren't staying in as peak of shape as they could be.

But it's different with the ears. There's really no muscle involved. We're really talking about neural stimulation. It's interesting. I have people who have struggled for years with poor hearing, who finally come in and decide to do something about it. They get hearing aids. They love their hearing aids. Maybe they come back to see me a year later and they go, "I take my hearing aids off. I don't hear anything without my hearing aids." I test their hearing and I say, "Your hearing hasn't changed over the last year. It's just that now, you have that immediate comparison of what it's like to hear well and then you take your hearing aids off at night and you can't hear anything. When it's gradual, you just deal with it. But when it's sudden, it's just so obvious."

JM: Oh. So what you're saying is that when a person comes in to get their hearing tested, I guess the word would be a baseline. Then they start treatment and they are enjoying the hearing aids. Then they come in for a follow-up. Kind of like you go to the dentist for a teeth cleaning, et cetera.

DSM: Yes.

JM: You come in and they say, "I can't hear anything without them," but you test them again. It's like taking an X-ray at the dentist. No, your teeth are still the way they were at our last cleaning. You're just enjoying the feeling of the cleaning.

DSM: Yes, that's exactly right. Now they have something to compare it to and it's a stark comparison.

JM: OK. Wow, that's interesting. I guess that makes sense. There really isn't any muscular involvement in the ears. It's because it's all vibration.

DSM: No.

JM: It's a response.

DSM: And it's surprising how many people I get in because the wife insists that the husband comes in for a test. He says, "I think I hear pretty well. I hear most of what I need to hear."

So then I put him in the booth. We test hm. We find he has a high frequency hearing loss. We put some hearing instruments on that just amplify the region that he's missing and he just brightens up and says, "Oh! I had no idea. Oh! Is this what everybody hears?"

Most people wait on average seven years from the time they first think they might have hearing loss. So by the time when they actually get hearing aids, they forget what crisp clean sound really sounds like. They think they're doing OK because they've developed all these adaptive behaviors. When you show them and let them experience what good hearing is like, then the heads start nodding and the smiles start coming on the faces. It's great work.

JM: Wow. It's obvious that you enjoy what you're doing.

Audio 4

JM: Welcome back. My guest today is Dr. Sunni McBride and we are talking about the importance of taking care of your hearing and before the break, we were talking about how I probably have some hearing loss and you're basically telling me to get over myself and have my hearing checked because you mentioned that if you're not hearing everything, you're not stimulating all the nerves in your brain and that it's actually changing your brain.

I was wondering if you could talk a little bit more about that. I mean it – can it affect your brain so much that you – it starts to affect other things in your mind?

DSM: Oh, absolutely. This is a recent research which has come out. Once again, remember the ear's job is to change sound waves into nerve impulses that will go up and stimulate your brain and specifically the auditory cortex on each side of your brain. So let's say you're in a noisy place and you're trying to figure out the conversation. Someone said, "Go get _______." So did they say, "Go get the cat?" Or "Go get the bat?" What did they say?

So you're thinking, "Well, let's see. We're talking about things at home, so they probably said CAT," and you do all these calculations instantaneously in your brain. You're just quickly trying to figure things out. When you are trying to figure out what somebody said, you're actually using a different part of your brain. It's the frontal part of your brain. If you put your hand right above your forehead...it's that part of your brain.

We don't have unlimited resources in our brain. It's what we call a closed system. It's similar to being on a budget. So if you only have so much money to spend and you're spending some of it to figure out what somebody said, then maybe you don't have enough money left for short-term memory or rapid computation or maintaining your balance or long working memory.

All these higher thinking processes that take brain energy, you're robbing them because you're taking some of that energy trying to figure out what someone said. We can actually measure it.

JM: Wow.

DSM: And there are standard tests of cognition. You take your mom to the neurologist and they have her draw a clock or they have her go through a worksheet that has 10 different questions and they time her and see what kind of different things she can remember, the days of the week backwards or whatever. They're standardized tests of cognition.

If you administer these tests to average people over time, you will find that in your 50s, you kind of have a baseline and then in your 60s, your brain starts to slow down and in your 70s, it slows down a little more and you can watch those scores slowly fall down.

Well, if you take a population with hearing loss, guess what. Those curves start sooner and they fall off faster.

JM: Wow.

DSM: So untreated hearing loss leads to a more rapid rate of cognitive decline. Do you understand that?

JM: Yeah, I do. That makes sense. Yeah.

DSM: And the scary thing is when we think about cognitive decline, what's at the end of that road is dementia and Alzheimer's and that's something that we are beginning to see as a national crisis in this country. As we have an aging population, the number of people with dementia and Alzheimer's is just continuing to climb.

The fascinating research coming out of Harvard associates hearing loss with developing dementia. The greater the hearing loss, the greater the probability of developing dementia.

In fact, they looked at huge populations of people with dementia. They tried to figure out what the risk factors were that will predict who will develop dementia. Then they lined them up in order of the most significant factors to the least significant factors. The number one modifiable risk factor for developing dementia is untreated hearing loss.

JM: Wow.

DSM: Isn't that fascinating?

JM: Yeah, it is. I never would have thought of that.

DSM: It correlates with dementia more than age, more than smoking, more than high blood pressure or a lack of nutrition or poor exercise. All of those things have less influence in the development of dementia than untreated hearing loss.

JM: So get your hearing checked.

DSM: It's a scary thought. But it's something that we can do something about. They currently have research that's undergoing that will be done in the next year or two where they're following populations to see the effect of hearing aids on people with hearing loss. So we cannot yet put the final dot at the end of the sentence. But at least we can try to do what we can to deal with hearing loss and dementia instead of trying to ignore it.

JM: Or at least pick up on the clues and use the information in a positive way as opposed to just kind of pretending that it might not help.

DSM: Right. And we need to change the conversation about hearing loss. What does hearing loss mean to you? I mean when you think of wearing a hearing aid, what does that mean to you?

JM: Me? It's like you're getting older.

DSM: Yes. You're not alone in feeling that way.

JM: I still mentally – I feel like I'm in my 20s. Anyway – and physically I feel really good too. So it's just like, well, that's an old person problem and I'm sorry.

DSM: That's right. So when people think of hearing aids, they think it will make them look old.

JM: Yeah.

DSM: Or broken. I hear people say, "Well, I can't let anybody at work see that I'm wearing a hearing aid. They won't promote me. They will think I'm less capable." So we need to change the conversation about what good hearing means.

JM: Well, for me, that's kind of a real thing. I mean if people are wondering whether or not I'm hearing things, well, they're saying, "Oh, how does this work?"

DSM: And it's so interesting. When I talk to people with hearing loss who wear hearing aids, they say, "I want people to see my hearing aid. I want them to know that I'm having a challenge because I want them to help me out."

JM: Oh, interesting.

DSM: And people who are successful hearing aid users are so joyful and grateful and delighted to be able to hear again and to hear with less energy and to have better images about themselves. They have better relationships. One thing that you don't realize is people with hearing loss tend to withdraw. Just think about yourself going into a party room and there are 50 people in there and they're all yakking and talking. The acoustics are terrible. Maybe the band is playing and you can only hear or understand half of what's being said.

JM: Yeah.

DSM: Are you going to walk right up to somebody and engage them in a conversation?

JM: Probably not. I would probably want to leave.

DSM: Yes. You probably want to leave because it's just too hard and frustrating to try to figure out what's going on. That's an extreme example. But people start not going to play bridge anymore because they can't follow it. Then peoples choose not to go to movies anymore because it's too hard to hear and they start making these little decisions in their lives. They start not being a part of the family conversation at the table because they can't follow it. So they just withdraw into a world of their own. That may not be the kind of person you used to be.

You probably were an outgoing person and to now live in this world of isolation, it's very sad and it begins to affect your overall health. As we slow down, withdraw and sit down, it affects our overall health.

Audio 5

JM: Welcome back. My guest today is Dr. Sunni McBride and we're talking about the importance of hearing and treating any kind of hearing loss and doctor, before the break, you were telling us about how hearing loss – we're finding out that it's a huge contributor or a high risk factor for leading to dementia.

You also mentioned that it can lead to other health problems. What kind of health problems are we talking about?

DSM: Well, there's a direct correlation between the degree of hearing loss that you have and your risk of falling. The greater the hearing loss, the greater the risk of falling. Now as you know, seniors are at risk for falling. Oftentimes if someone falls and breaks a hip, only 50 percent of those people will be alive a year later. So falls are extremely debilitating and cause a huge expense to our country.

Aside from that, you can kind of think of the isolation that is caused by hearing loss, which causes people to retreat and retire and slow down. Your life becomes smaller and smaller instead of wild and crazy, like your life is now. You're active and doing all these things. As you become smaller and smaller with the activities that you do, your blood pressure changes. Your musculature changes. All these changes take place.

So that's kind of directly related to what hearing loss causes. But another interesting thing to consider is what causes hearing loss. We've talked about noise and external factors. But sometimes people think hearing loss may be the canary in the coal mine for other diseases in your body.

Miners used to put canaries in the coal mine because when the gas is starting to get bad, the canaries would keel over before the miners did. So it was kind of a signal that something was going wrong. Well, when you start having hearing loss, it could be a sign of kidney disease. It could be a sign of heart disease. Hearing loss and diabetes are extremely closely related. Insulin resistance in the body, everything that causes what we call metabolic syndrome, you know, resistance to insulin, development of diabetes and heart disease, it all affects the fine blood vessels that go up into the ear.

JM: Wow.

DSM: So if you have any of these other diseases, you probably have hearing loss and hearing loss can be a sign that these other diseases are taking place.

JM: Fascinating. So it could be – yeah. So hearing loss could be symptomatic of other underlying problems.

DSM: Yes.

JM: Fascinating. Wow. Are there any other conditions that hearing loss can create?

DSM: Sure. There's a condition that's very prevalent in the population called tinnitus. Tinnitus refers to ringing sounds in your ear or buzzing or chirping. It's phantom sounds that you perceive in your head that really aren't there. But you hear them. A lot of people, especially when they go to sleep at night, they start hearing a ringing in their ears. It can be anything from intermittent and mild to severe, loud, unrelenting head noises that you just feel like you can't escape from.

It's interesting when you do the research. About 80 percent of people who have tinnitus also have hearing loss. An audiologist in our clinic just told me this week about a patient that he saw that has had ringing in the ears for 10 years. He had been to eight ear, nose and throat doctors. It's just driving him crazy. He came to see us. We found out he had hearing loss. We put some demonstration hearing aids on him and made sure they were finally tuned in the regions where his tinnitus was occurring and the audiologist was talking to him and said, "So are you hearing it now?"

The guy looked up into his head and listened and was about in tears. He says, "This is the first time in 10 years that I haven't heard my tinnitus."

JM: Wow.

DSM: It's just amazing. So tinnitus is a phantom sound. If you have hearing loss in a certain area, those nerves that are supposed to be firing through stimulation from sound waves really aren't firing. They're just sitting there and the nerve chemicals where the nerves join together, they're creating their own neural energy. It's almost like when you listen to a seashell. There's no sound in there but you kind of hear something. It's similar to veterans with amputee pain.

JM: OK.

DSM: Unfortunately, tinnitus can be devastating. One of my father's friends that went through medical school with him was so bothered by tinnitus. He actually founded the American Tinnitus Association many years ago and devoted his life's work to it. Tinnitus is so disturbing, it has led some people to suicide.

So when we see tinnitus patients in our clinic, we want to do a thorough evaluation. Sometimes it's just caused by hearing loss. Tinnitus can be caused by medication. It can be caused by poor jaw alignment of the TMJ joint. If you have TMJ problems, that can cause tinnitus. There are lots of things that cause tinnitus. So between your medical doctor and your audiologist, we really try to identify the cause of your tinnitus. Is it just a hearing problem or is it something else?

We do a lot of education. If you have tinnitus and you compound it with worry and anxiety and OCD, that can take a physical problem and spin it into something more because of the emotional energy that you give to it. So by focusing in on your tinnitus and going, "Oh my gosh. I think it's louder today. It's louder in the right ear than the left. I don't know if I can do this," by doing that self-talk, you're actually making it seem louder in your head.

JM: Wow.

DSM: We do counseling . We do testing. We do therapy either using hearing aids or other sound generators and we try to bring that emotional level back and unwind it and stimulate the brain in an appropriate way. We have been able to help most of the people that have come through our door, with their tinnitus. It's a great blessing in their lives.

JM: That's amazing. We have to take another break. But I am so fascinated by this topic. I want to talk to you about – we've talked about all the things that can cause hearing loss and some of the other health risks associated with hearing loss and how hearing loss can be a symptom of other health risks. So we've painted a picture as to how important it is for people to get their hearing checked and their hearing loss treated.

When we come back, can we talk about the treatment and some of the changes that happen as a result of getting your hearing loss treated?

DSM: Sure, that will be fun.

Audio 6

JM: Welcome back. My guest today is Dr. Sunni McBride and we are talking about hearing loss and hearing loss treatments and doctor, I want to thank you for spending so much time with us today. I am learning a lot and I know our audience is learning a lot as well. So thank you for sharing your information with us.

DSM: Happy to do it.

JM: So just before our last break, you were talking about tinnitus, the ringing in the ears and how some hearing aids or maybe all of them, I don't know, have helped people get rid of their tinnitus or make it so that they can't hear it anymore. It sounds like pretty amazing technology that these hearing aids are able to treat that problem and some of the other problems that you're talking about today. How big a role is technology playing in hearing loss these days?

DSM: That's what makes it so fun to be an audiologist today. If you think about how computers have changed over the last 10, 15 years, I mean what is it? The iPhone has only been out for 10 years.

JM: Yeah.

DSM: Well, the same kind of computer change and development has been occurring in hearing instruments. I've been to several of the international manufacturers and been through their plants and seen the design of circuit boards from when they had four transistors on the board to now they have 30 million transistors in a single hearing aid. It has just become so complicated engineering-wise. But the results for the end user are so marvelous.

When I first got into hearing aids, they still had old-fashioned hearing aids that you adjusted with a screwdriver. Somebody would say, "I don't really like the sound." You had two screwdriver heads in there that you could crank a little bit. "Here, try that. Is that any better?" Crank it the other way. "Well, how about that? How does that sound?"

So literally, I had two things to adjust in a hearing aid and now with digital circuits – I used to say there are 40 things I can adjust. Now there are even more ways to adjust them. They're so complex. They're just so fluid. The technology has been marvelous.

So let's talk about tinnitus and technology. Once again, that ringing in the ears. You take a hearing instrument and if you see a good audiologist who really measures the sound coming out of a hearing aid right while it sits in your ear, they can map it to exactly match your hearing loss. When you stimulate those frequencies, the tinnitus starts to fade. Additionally, they can have a tinnitus sound generator program built into the hearing aid.

Some people have white noise fans that they turn on by their bed at night or maybe they have a sound generator by their bed that emits the sounds of babbling brooks or wind in the trees. Now they've developed something like that built into the hearing aid. So maybe you're just wearing your hearing aid all day long because you have hearing loss and you go home. It's really quiet. Nobody is around, not like your house I'm sure, and they want to sit on there and read the paper.

Well, that's a time when their tinnitus would be really loud because it's really quiet. So then they just click a button on their hearing aid and it turns on this kind of white noise, ocean-like sound, coming and going. It doesn't cover up your tinnitus. It gives your brain something else to pay attention to.

So your brain is not really focusing in on that ringing sound of your head. Once again, the less your brain focuses on that sound, the less attention it gives to it, the more it tends to fade into the background, right?

JM: Interesting.

DSM: So hearing aids with sound generators have been found to be more effective than a hearing aid alone. Then if you take it to the next level, there is a relatively new device called the Lyric Extended Wear hearing instrument. This is a hearing instrument that was developed at the University of San Francisco 11 or 12 years ago. It's a totally unique hearing instrument. There's only one like it on the planet. It's yellow because it's made out of yellow compressible foam. The compressible foam encircles the battery and electronic core to cushion it, making it comfortable in your ear.

So it makes it just a really small little comfortable device that we try to insert deep in your ear canal about four millimeters from the eardrum. That hearing aid, the Lyric Extended Hearing Aid Device, stays in your ear day and night until the battery dies, which is about two to three months.

From a wearing point of view, it's kind of like wearing an extended wear contact lens. You put it in and you forget about it. But if you think about it, you're hearing amplified sound in your ear day and night.

Now I know you think you go to sleep at night and your brain goes to sleep. But it doesn't. While you're sleeping at night, your brain is on overload doing all sorts of regenerative processes. If while you're sleeping at night you've got Lyric in and it's hearing cars going by, it's hearing ticking clocks, it's hearing your partner snore, you're still getting stimulated all night long. Lyric has been shown to be the most effective tool for helping tinnitus to fade fastest because you've got that stimulation 24/7.

JM: Oh, interesting. That's fascinating.

DSM: Isn't that amazing?

JM: Yeah. So do you feel it inside there? Sometimes you get an itchy ear and you want to scratch your ear and all that kind of stuff. Does it interfere with itching your ears?

Audio 7

DSM: I bet you love to clean your ears with Q-tips too, don't you?

JM: I don't. No. I know that's a bad thing. I know that's –

DSM: OK, good. Your mother taught you well.

JM: Yeah. Nothing smaller than your elbow is what she told me.

DSM: Right, very good.

JM: Yeah.

DSM: Yes, a lot of people have itchy ears and you can still fit the Lyric. It comes with seven different sizes. It doesn't fit in every ear. But if you can get it properly placed, comfortably fit – I have patients who just say, "I forget I'm wearing it. I don't even feel it anymore."

JM: Wow.

DSM: Those are the patients that just love their Lyric. It's great quality sound. They like not having to fiddle with batteries. They never have to take it in and out of their ears. It's great for people with dementia, who would never remember to put a hearing aid on.

In fact I tell caregivers for dementia people, "You are going to love this because once we put this in your ears, you don't have to worry about it." When one of the hearing aids dies, the demented person probably won't remember to tell you, "Oh, you know what? I think my hearing aid died." But when two of them die, you're going to know it because you can't talk to this person anymore. The Lyrics become very effective ear plugs.

JM: Oh, OK.

DSM: When the Lyrics are dead, then you come back to our office. We take them out. We throw them away. We make sure your ear is free of wax. We program some new Lyrics, put them in your ears and say, "See you in two to three months."

JM: Wow.

DSM: So it's carefree use for two to three months with an occasional visit back to our office. It's really a fun product.

JM: Ha! That's fascinating. So there are all kinds of different hearing aids, right?

DSM: Certainly. The Lyric, as I said, is the only extended wear hearing aid that stays in your ear. But there are small hearing aids that can be custom-molded to your ear. They don't go in as deep as the Lyric does. The Lyric is totally invisible.

You can also get a custom-molded hearing aid that's invisible. But there are some trade-offs. You have to take that little teeny-weeny hearing aid out every day. If your fingers aren't good, that might be a problem. Teeny-weeny hearing aids have teeny-weeny batteries. That can be a problem and they don't last very long. Your ear is kind of like a swamp. It's kind of warm and moist and humid and guess where all that moisture goes. It goes right into the teeny-weeny hearing aid.

So these invisible down-in-your-ear hearing aids sometimes require more repairs, more cleaning, things like that. But if you're a person who says, "Hey, it has got to be invisible," then Lyric or the small custom-made hearing aids are the option.

I say everything has a trade-off in hearing aids. When you first show someone a hearing instrument that actually sits behind their ear, external to their ear and has a little wire coming down the front with a piece that goes inside, some people initially say, "I don't know if I want something that people can see."

JM: Yeah.

DSM: But then when you put it on and you show them that just a little small rubber tip is going in their ear canal, they say that they hardly feel it at all. Then you tell them that this has rechargeable batteries. When you take them off your ears at night, you just drop them into the recharger. They recharge overnight. Put them on again. You don't have to change batteries every two or three days. Well, that becomes a little more appealing to people, right?

JM: Right, yeah.

DSM: And then when you say, "Now with your iPhone, we're going to connect your iPhone to your hearing aid!" A lot of people with hearing challenges have trouble understanding on their cell phone. Even with hearing aids, some might still have trouble understanding on their cell phone.

Now with modern hearing aids, you can pair your hearing aid directly to the iPhone. When that phone rings and you push the little green button to answer the call, the voice goes into both of your ears at the same time perfectly clearly.

JM: That's fascinating.

DSM: Yes. And the brain loves having sound in two ears compared to one. A lot more chance to understand what's being said. You can control the volume. It's not a speaker phone. Nobody else can hear it. It's like wearing your own personal ear buds.

JM: Interesting.

DSM: But you don't have to put anything on. It's just in your hearing aids that you're wearing all day long.

JM: That's fascinating. You're probably not yelling into the phone because –

DSM: It's so easy to hear.

JM: Yeah.

DSM: And any sound that comes out of that iPhone, whether it's FaceTime or YouTube videos or Pandora music or an Audible book, all you have to do is get it started. It's right in your hearing aid. You can put your phone in your pocket and go for a bike ride or go for a walk. You've got direct audio input in your hearing aid.

JM: That's amazing. Who would have thought it? This doesn't sound like the stuff that you can see on the television and some of the ads in the brochures that you get in the mail.

DSM: Correct.

JM: We need to talk about that when we come back. OK?

Audio 8

JM: Welcome back. My guest today is Dr. Sunni McBride and we're talking about hearing loss, hearing treatment and hearing technology. Doctor, before the break, you were telling me some really neat things about some of the technology for treating hearing loss. Not all of them but some of them, some of these new high-tech devices.

So it's almost like your own personal ear buds along with being able to hear everything else.

DSM: Yes. We call it streaming. It uses low energy Bluetooth to stream directly into the hearing aids. You can even get devices that you can plug into your television set that convert the audio signal in the television set to a low energy Bluetooth signal, that will also stream directly to your hearing aids.

Some people get amplified headphones or TV ears that they put on every night when they want to watch TV. You don't have to do that anymore. If you have these streaming hearing aids, you just push a button and all of a sudden, you've got the voices inside of your head.

JM: I've got voices inside of my head too. But not from these technology gizmos! But I do want to ask you. You know, there seems to be so much advertising about hearing devices. You know, like you can hear people secretly talking about you from across the room and the brochures that you get in the mail and the other things that – you know: call now and we will double your order type stuff. We're not talking about that, are we?

DSM: Right. No. And mail-order hearing aids have been around for decades. There used to be the Crystal Ear. You could buy out of the Parade magazine for $25.

JM: Yeah, yeah.

DSM: And I think they just figured that people weren't going to return it. They just throw it in the trash and so those people made millions of dollars, trying to entice people to do something. Hearing aids today are such sophisticated devices. But there's a lot of competition in the field, a lot of consumer electronic people like Samsung and other companies. They want to get into the business. They see this growing population of baby boomers. If you look at the statistics of the percentage of people with hearing loss, how many of those actually get hearing help through hearing aids? Right now, there's only about a 20 percent penetration of the market.

JM: Wow.

DSM: So you could double or triple the number of hearing aid users just right now and you wouldn't fill the whole market. Then when you see how the aging baby boomers are going to double the amount of people with hearing loss in the next decade or so, I mean everybody is just salivating at the thought of all of this.

So what's going to happen? There are going to be people who feel like they have to compete on price. So they're going to come out with cheap hearing aids that don't have great technology. They're going to be kind of a do-it-yourself. One-size-fits-all with 3 basic settings you can try. You try it and you put it in your ear and maybe you think it helps you and great.

My question is if something is not fit properly, how is it going to help you? How effective is it going to be? How do you know what good sound is? Your hearing has deteriorated for the last 10 years. You don't know what normal sound is supposed to be like. Is there a risk of putting too much sound in your ears and ruining it further? There certainly is.

JM: Yeah.

DSM: When we sell hearing aids to people, we want them to come back to our office. We want to monitor their experience. We want to clean and test those hearing aids periodically because guess what, they're just digital, electronic devices. Over time, they're going to break down. We know hearing goes down. Hearing aids break down. They get clogged with wax. If you don't have a local audiologist, who are you going to take it to when it's not working right?

There was one insurance company that was working with a company and you mail them a copy of your hearing test and they mail you your hearing aids. It has three typical settings. Maybe one of them might be somewhat close to what you might need and if you have a problem, then you mail it back to them.

That is not they type of service that most of my patients want and need. I have so many people that sit in my chair and we work with them and we show them how to use their devices. We practice putting them on their ears. They come back for a follow up and tell us that somethings might be a little too loud or a little too soft. We go in and fine-tune and shape the sound. Maybe your hearing changes over time. We go in and we change it again. It takes professional time and energy and care to make someone successful. It's completely different than buying a pair of shoes or reader glasses where you find something that fits and then you are done.

Even with traditional hearing aids, there are different technology levels that come in similar looking body styles. So maybe the most basic technology hearing aid sells for $1200 for one and maybe the top end of their technology sells for $3500 for one. Is there a difference in how you're going to perform and how you're going to perceive sound? Absolutely. Like most things in life, you get what you pay for.

JM: Yeah. A couple of things have popped into my head as you were telling me this. If you've got one of those devices that you're supposed to mail back for tune-ups and such, how does that help you hear? I mean how long are you going to be without them? The other thing is, is based on all of the health implications, not just your hearing but mental health and your physical health, the heart disease and things of that nature that you mentioned, are all tied into hearing.

It just seems to make sense to me that you don't want to just trust all those other factors to a $29.95 speaker, right?

DSM: Right. When someone comes to me and I do a full audiological evaluation, we have what we call the red flag questions. Have you experienced dizziness, ringing in your ears? Is it one ear or both? Any sudden changes in your hearing? Sudden onset of ringing? Do you have ear pain? Do you have drainage? All these things we ask them because maybe it's not plain old vanilla hearing loss.

Maybe there's something medically going on in your head, in your ears. We've talked about noise-related hearing loss. But a hearing loss could be caused anywhere from wax in your ears to a perforated ear drum. Or the three little bones behind it, the hammer, anvil and stirrup, can begin to calcify together. Those kinds of things can be fixed by surgery. Maybe you don't even need a hearing aid.

JM: Wow.

DSM: Maybe you have a health condition that's going on and on that should be medically treated. Unfortunately, you could even have a tumor growing on the nerve that connects your ear up to the brain.

JM: Wow.

DSM: If you don't know the signs of what to look for, you might live for years with that. If you go to an audiologist and they test it and they start to see some of these red flags, well then we know we have to medically refer you for follow-up care.

But if you're taking care of yourself, it's kind of like people who ignore lumps on their breasts or other signs. They just kind of ignore it until it's too late.

JM: Yeah.

DSM: It's interesting. The FDA has had very strong consumer protection laws built into their regulations over the last few decades and now with this rush of, "Oh my! Hearing aids are so expensive. We need to lower the cost, so everybody can have them. So we will just flood the market with whatever and they can take care of themselves," they're just eliminating all the consumer protection laws that they've enacted.

JM: Oh, that's interesting.

DSM: It's really sad to see the pressure that is being put on the FDA by these consumer electronics and other groups. It's interesting. This gets into politics and things but everybody thinks the number one reason people don't wear hearing aids is because they cost too much.

Well, they've done studies. They go to places like Japan and other countries where the government will pay 100 percent for hearing aids and guess what, the market penetration isn't any higher than it is in the United States.

JM: Oh, that's interesting.

DSM: Why? Because people feel like you do. "I don't want a hearing aid."

JM: Yeah.

DSM: It makes me feel old and broken and weird and I don't want to.

JM: Yeah. You're using me against myself. No, that's fine.

DSM: They do surveys of hearing aid users. Every year, there's an organization that for decades now has been doing customer surveys to try to figure out attitudes and trends, and when they ask people about their resistance to hearing aids, price is not the number one issue. It's way down on the list.

So we're afraid they're going to cause a lot of unintended consequences under the guise of trying to do good.

JM: Oh, yeah. Well, how many times has that happened?

DSM: Well, right, exactly. So we in the business, we feel like cheap hearing aids have always been available. If you want a cheap hearing aid right now, you can go get a hearing aid for $350 or $750. You get what you pay for. But if that's what you want, it's available right now. For people who try those things, it's fine. If it amplifies sound, helps you a little bit, fine. When you get to the point that you say, "I really still can't understand speech when there is background noise. This really doesn't help me in soft-speech situations," then maybe it's time to go seek a professional and get real professional care. We like to take the hard cases. We like to take the ones that aren't fixed by easy, quick fixes. We feel there will always be people out there who need us and we will be there for them.

JM: That sounds good. You know, I have to take another break. But when we come back, let's talk about how to choose somebody to help treat your hearing loss.

DSM: OK.

Audio 9

JM: Welcome back. My guest today has been Dr. Sunni McBride and we've been talking about treating hearing loss, the technology that goes into treating hearing loss and we've been talking about how you can get some cheap stuff through the magazines and all that. But really, if you want something that's going to serve you well, I guess is a good way to put it, then you really do need to make an investment in high quality hearing devices.

But the other question I wanted to ask you doctor was – we talked about how if you want to spend 300 bucks on a pair of hearing devices, then that's your choice. But if you really want to improve your hearing, improve your overall health, your mental health and physical health, you should go seek professional treatment. How does somebody go about finding the right person to treat their hearing loss?

DSM: Yes, that's really important to find the right person. As I said, this is not a one-time experience. You're going to be developing a relationship with this person over time. You're making an investment on something that you're going to wear on your body every day for the next three to five years. So if you think about it that way, then it kind of gives it some perspective.

So we really recommend that you get someone who's a trained specialist, a doctor of audiology or a licensed hearing instrument specialist who has had a lot of experience. With the exploding population, CVS is going to try to put a hearing center in every store and big box stores have hearing centers.

Just because they could sell tires or diapers really well doesn't mean that they should necessarily sell hearing aids now. It takes training to understand how the ear works and to understand how hearing works and sound and electronics and how it all interacts.

My new audiologists that I'm hiring now have four-year degrees after college. So they've been in school for eight years learning about this stuff.

JM: Wow.

DSM: And even audiologists. There are some that are more careful, some that are more caring. You can have an initial visit. You know, look on their website and read their bios. Look at their degrees. Look at the reviews in particular to see how do people act with these people in the office.

You should consider. Is it a medical office or is it just a hearing aid office? You want someone who has some depth behind what they do. Are they aware of the brain issues with hearing or are they just trying to sell you a device?

JM: Right.

DSM: We use very specialized equipment to measure the output of the hearing aid while it sits in your ear. Consumer reports said 60 percent of the hearing aids that they surveyed were not adjusted properly.

JM: Sixty percent?

DSM: Sixty percent.

JM: Oh my goodness.

DSM: And I think that's because most people grew up in an era where you put it on a patient and you would say, "Well, how does that sound?" Well, I think I need it a little louder. All right. We will turn things up. How does that sound? Well, it seems a little tinny. OK. Well, I will move these little buttons and supposedly it moves things down. Does that sound better? So you're just going by subjective feel of the patient.

What we do is we make objective measurements. We have a little probe tube. We put it in the ear right next to the hearing device.

We can exactly measure the speech sounds coming out of that device through a program and we can match it to your hearing loss.

JM: That's fascinating.

DSM: We make changes on the computer. We can see the changes that it's making in the hearing aid. Sometimes you can push those buttons all you want and it's really not changing anything. You watch the numbers on your graph go up really pretty in the hearing aid software. When you measure in the ear, it's not changing for some reason or another. If you don't measure it, you don't know.

So you really have to ask, "Do they do real ear measurements or live speech mapping?" Those are the two most accurate ways of figuring out what the hearing aids are doing in your ear. A lot of people don't have the equipment or don't take the time or don't have knowledge to do that.

JM: I hate to say it this way. But is that why they cost so much, because of this technology?

DSM: Well, you have to understand at least with our office, when you buy a hearing aid from us, you're not just buying the widget. You are buying all of our service and care. Everything that you need for the next three years to be successful is included, however many visits you need during that time. As I say, we want people to come in for routine cleanings and acoustic evaluations of their hearing aids. We give them batteries. We are full service people.

When you walk in the door after you've bought our hearing aid, we don't ask you to get your wallet out and cough up money again. We say, "Welcome. What do you need today?" and we take care of it. Some people look for the cheapest price of a hearing aid on the internet. OK? So first, you need to know that most major manufacturers do not allow internet sales. If manufacturers find out anybody is ordering hearing aids and selling them on the internet, they will shut them down and revoke their ability to sell their products.

JM: Dealership thing, yeah. Wow.

DSM: So the manufacturers, the international manufacturers, understand that it takes a professional to make their products work right. But even so, there are different brands and things that you can buy on the internet and they think, "OK. Well, I got it a lot cheaper than I can get it from you." OK. Well, who's going to take care of you now, when you have a problem?

JM: Right.

DSM: Oh, can I just pay for one visit? It takes more than one visit to make hearing aids work right over the next three years. So we used to kind of do what we call "un-bundle our services," where, "Sure. OK. We will charge you. When you want your hearing aid cleaned, it will be this much. OK. You want this done. It will be this much." You know – and it's like nickel-and-diming of people. Then what happens is people think, "Well, I really should get that tuned up. But I don't think I want to pay for it right now. So I will skip it."

JM: Yeah.

DSM: And then their hearing aid is not working very well. So it's just a can of worms.

JM: Yeah.

DSM: So we just decided. We know what it takes to make people successful. We deliver on the service promise that we make. Some people, they just want to move on to the next sale. They don't want you coming back. They don't want to service you. They don't want to take the time because they're on to the next sale. That's not who we are. That's not how we work.

JM: It's kind of like if you get on the airplane and then they give you a deal on the seat and then if you want more leg room, you got to pay X amount. Then if you want food, you got to pay a little bit more and if you want to watch the movie, then it's another four bucks and all that kind. So just add $10 on to the cost of the ticket and just include it and it's a lot less.

DSM: Exactly. I think people don't want to be nickel-and-dimed.

JM: Yeah, that makes sense. You break that out over the course of a year, it's probably dollars a day.

DSM: Another thing that you need to consider is what kind of technology are they providing. Once again, something you're going to invest in to wear on your body every day for the next three to five years. Do you want the latest technology that's available and the very best bet we can come up with or do you want something that was the best four years ago? I mean it was good then. Maybe it's good enough or would you really rather have something that performs the best. How many people are going back and buying iPhone 5 right now? Not too many people, right?

JM: That's true, yeah.

DSM: If you're going to invest that much money, you want the best functionality because you are more likely to be successful and to be comfortable with what you're wearing. So we just deal with the five major manufacturers in the world and we deal with their top technology products. I really don't sell Medi-Cal quality hearing aids, the dumbed-down, simplified cheap hearing aids. It's just a lot more work for us.

JM: Yeah.

DSM: People who have purchased cheap hearing aids come back to us and say, "I still can't hear." Really? The background noise is really loud because you don't have any technology in the hearing aid to help suppress the background noise. So I'm sorry. They are inexpensive because they are just amplifiers. It's a no-win situation. So we try to deal with technology that will help people and move them forward and help them to be successful.

So hearing aids may look alike. But if it's not the latest technology, then you're overpaying for something and not getting the best that's available.

JM: That's fascinating. That just makes sense really in the long run. I need to take another break. But when we come back, let's talk about your practice specifically and how people can learn more about South Bay Hearing. OK?

DSM: OK.

Audio 10

JM: Welcome back. My guest today is Dr. Sunni McBride and we're talking about hearing wellness, if you will. We're talking about hearing loss and hearing treatment and technology, and Doctor, this has been a great conversation. I have learned so much today about all the implications of hearing loss.

It's not that you're just not hearing well. But it can lead to dementia, other health risks, social isolation, and insecurity and all of that and it affects everybody in the family and your friends. Hearing loss has wide-ranging effects. We've talked about the technology that's now available to help treat hearing loss and why it's probably worth the investment in this technology and that you shouldn't cheap out on it just because you're trying to save a buck because it's going to cost you more time and money in the long run anyway.

But one thing that we really haven't talked about too much is your practice at South Bay Hearing. So talk to us about that. How can people who want to learn more about your services do so? Tell us a little about your practice.

DSM: I would be happy to. So probably the best way to get a window into our practice is to go to our website which is www.SouthBayHearing.com. There you can get a feel for who we are and what we're about. We started this business in 2007. I've grown from myself and a secretary to now a staff of 5 doctors of audiology and a staff of 12 people to assist us here and a second office in Mission Viejo. When I opened my business, I had this vision in my mind that I wanted to make the patient experience different from any other experience they would have looking for hearing aids anywhere in the South Bay.

So it starts with the phone calls and the voice at the end of the line and how helpful they can be and how welcoming they can be. When you walk in our doors, we want it to be warm and inviting and we want our staff to just wrap their arms around you and suck you in.

My husband used to laugh. He worked with me and he said, "You know, I don't know what you do back there." He said, "I watch people walk in from the parking lot and they're frowning and they're unhappy and they come in. By the time they spend an hour and a half with you, they come out and they're laughing and they're happy."

JM: Wow. An hour and a half, that's unheard of.

DSM: That's what we spend with a new patient because it takes that much time to really get to know you and your needs, to thoroughly evaluate your hearing, to show you your options, to let you actually experience good hearing. We demonstrate hearing aids on everyone.

You will know exactly what it feels like to hear good again. It's a life-changing experience for people. So we want to change fear and uncertainty into confidence. We educate people. My feeling is an educated patient is better able to make good decisions for themselves. I try to lay out all the options and kind of walk them through that process to show them what's important in making a decision.

You go look at a car and you can look at 0 to 60 times and you can look at breaking distances. It's a little harder to kick the tires with a hearing aid. It's a much more subjective experience and there are lots of subjective factors that go into picking the right hearing instrument for you. So we really want to spend the time and do that.

I love my staff. They are so warm and welcoming. I have one staff member who will walk up to somebody and say, "You look like you need a hug today," and give them a hug.

We send out birthday cards and invite people to come in to get their little birthday gift, which is usually some free batteries and some chocolates or something. Then my staff puts on their party hats and kazoos "Happy Birthday to You."

JM: Really?

DSM: Yes. I mean it's a fun place. We deal with a lot of senior people who don't have a lot going on in their life sometimes. I mean we have people that say, "This means so much to me. You're the only people who remembered my birthday."

We want you to come back. We want you to be a part of our family. When I hire my audiologists, I look for the top professionals that I can find. We run a busy place around here. You have to like people. You have to be smart. You have to know how to work with people and you have to know how to work together as a team.

Now if you can't do that, then this isn't really the right place for you. We are so involved in our customer care. The patient comes first. We always try to solve problems with the patient in mind and I think we can kind of see the results. Our reviews on Google have skyrocketed. We have our local newspaper,

The Daily Breeze. We've been voted the Best Audiologists in our community for the last 10 years in a row.

JM: Wow.

DSM: It's just the readers supporting and voting for us. So we're really appreciative of them. We try to provide top technology. We're the only providers of the Lyric Extended Wear hearing aid in the South Bay. Actually I think south of Beverly Hills probably. We're one of the largest Lyric offices in the country. I've actually traveled nationally and internationally lecturing on how to use Lyrics effectively. They would open up a country like Holland or the Netherlands and train people there and then about six months later, I would come in and work with individual practice owners to say, "OK. Now you've been doing this for a while. Tell me all your questions because guess what, we've had the same questions and we know how to work through the problems."

So it has been fun. It's fun to lecture, to meet people around the world and that we're able to bring that expertise back to our office and help our patients. We invite people to come and see us. I think you will be surprised when you walk through the door. You will certainly feel welcome and we will do the best that we can to help you out.

JM: You know, it looks like we've got a phone call coming in. Let's go ahead and take that.

Audio 11

JM: Hi. Welcome to the program. Who's calling please?

P: My name is Mike West.

JM: Hi Mike. How are you today?

P: I'm doing great. Thank you.

JM: Are you a patient of Dr. McBride's?

P: Yes, I am.

JM: What prompted you to go see her and what was your experience like?

P: Well, my wife had been encouraging me to go see an audiologist for a while and we joked about the old joke about, "I don't need a hearing aid. I have a hearing aid. It's called my wife." That wore out after a while and so Dr. McBride's office has a good local reputation. We looked her up online. So we decided to go see her. But I was pretty blown away with the amount of technology that's used in the hearing aids today and particularly in her office.

JM: How so?

P: Well, first of all, she gave me a hearing test, which is in a little booth and you press a button when you hear some noises. But after that, she has got this big screen, like a monitor up on the wall that showed where my hearing losses were and which frequencies and then she pulled out a couple of hearing aids and through Bluetooth, all the information from my hearing test was downloaded into these two hearing aids.

She made some small adjustments. In a pretty quick order, she had a pair for me to try on. She said most of my hearing loss is in the higher frequencies. So she said, "I'm not going to set these hearing aids to normal because you haven't been hearing high frequencies for a long time. So I think it's going to be a little bit too much for you. So I'm going to reduce it to about 20 percent."

Hearing aids were programmed for my hearing loss and each individual frequency. It wasn't just like an overall volume up or down. It was specifically fine-tuned where I am deficient and it would raise it where I was normal and didn't touch it.

JM: Wow.

P: I said OK. So she quickly downloaded all the information from her computer through Bluetooth into the two hearing aids and put them on and said, "Well, let's go outside the office," you know, and like towards the main street that she's on. Walked out there and I was just sort of overwhelmed by the amount of activity and noise. It just sort of floored me even though my hearing aids were set lower. So she said, "It's going to take you a while after 20 years of not hearing these high frequencies for your brain to adjust. But your brain will adjust. In about two weeks, you should be ready for me to set the levels back to normal hearing," and that's exactly what happened.

So two weeks later, I came back and she boosted them up to normal levels and I can't live without them. It has been a life-changing experience. So I've gone in for some tune-ups and actually upgraded to a new one about a year ago. Hearing aid technologies are like smart phones. New and cool stuff comes out every year.

JM: Yeah.

P: That was my initial experience. I've been a happy client ever since.

JM: That's great. What would you say to someone who's getting the same messages that you were getting from family and friends? You know, you should get your hearing checked and they're going, "Yeah, yeah, yeah." What would you tell them?

P: I would say it's a free hearing test. So it doesn't cost anything to go on there and to do it. So why not? It's interesting. I've had these hearing aids for a while and every once in a while, the topic of hearing aids will come up and so I say, "Well, I have hearing aids." Some people I've known for a long time, I take them off the back from my ear and show them, and they say, "Man, I had no idea. I couldn't see anything."

JM: Yeah.

P: So some people are concerned about that. But the ability to hear conversations and – you know, I noticed that when my wife and I were watching TV programs or watching a Netflix show, I always had to have the subtitles on, so I could follow what was going on because my wife got tired of me saying, "What did they say?"

JM: Yeah. I'm laughing because I do the same thing.

P: Yeah. So I don't have to have subtitles anymore. I just listen to it. It's pretty great.

JM: That's awesome.

P: Yes, I would encourage people to go. The technology is new every year, they make these tremendous advances. So, I've asked her to keep me updated and if something new and better comes along, I'm going to go there and get it, although I'm today completely satisfied.

JM: Well, that's wonderful. Mike, thank you for taking some time and sharing your thoughts with us today. I really appreciate it.

P: You bet. I'm happy to call in and talk to you. Thanks John.

JM: Is there anything else you can think of that you would like to share?

P: Yes, there's a short story about my grandfather. My grandfather lived to be 102 years old and when he was like in his 40s, he worked at a sheet metal shop and it was loud and noisy equipment. He had a significant hearing loss through much of my life. So there is the age difference between my grandfather and myself. So as a teenager and as a young adult, getting to know him that – I didn't really know him very well. We got together in family groups, for dinners and Sunday dinners and I would try to speak with him. Because of his hearing loss, I really didn't get to know him very well.

I just can't help but think what my relationship might have been like with my grandfather and how much closer we could have been if this technology was available in his time.

JM: Wow.

P: So I've got grandkids now. So I'm excited that I'm able to hear and understand and have detailed conversations with them. So because of technology, I'm going to be able to have a better relationship with my grandchildren than my grandfather did with me. It's an amazing, wonderful miracle!

JM: That's a very powerful story, Mike, and yeah, that's very touching and I want to thank you for sharing that.

P: You bet. Glad to.

Audio 12

JM: Well, doctor, they sound absolutely thrilled.

DSM: Oh, thank you. Yes. We love our patients and I'm glad they feel it.

JM: That's great. You mentioned that you're the only providers of the Lyric hearing aids in South Bay and even in your part of the Los Angeles area.

DSM: Yes. We're privileged to be the Lyric provider here in the South Bay area and it has been a good tool for us to use in our practice. We also are opening up the only hearing aid service center in Los Angeles. We've built out the space next door to us to build a lab. We're going to invite anyone, wherever they purchased their hearing aids, to come in. If they want to have them checked and cleaned onsite, we will do that. We can do minor repairs on site. If they need to be sent out to manufacturers, we can help them do that.

So this will be something totally new for our area. Once again, a hearing aid is only as good as it can be maintained. So we want to add that next level of service to our practice.

JM: You don't have to be a current patient of yours to take advantage of this service center?

DSM: No. You will be able to come in. Of course our patients will get the service free of charge. There may be a minor fee for our time and service. Sometimes it's hard to get into places to get the repairs or cleanings that you need. We want to make this easy for people to access.

JM: Oh, that's great. It looks like we have another phone call coming in. Let's go ahead and take that. Hi. Welcome to the program. Who's calling please?

P: Hi. This is Patty Hedrick.

JM: Hi Patty. How are you today?

P: I'm great. How about yourself?

JM: Very well, thank you. Are you a patient of Dr. McBride's?

P: Yes, I am.

JM: What was your experience like? Why did you go see her?

P: Well, I went to see her because I'm young, but everybody kept telling me that I couldn't hear them. So I went and got evaluated and ended up needing a hearing aid for one ear. It was hard for me because I never thought I was at the point that I needed a hearing aid. But they made everything wonderful and the hearing aid has made a huge difference in my life.

JM: I work in a studio. I deal with sound all day long and I'm wondering – I will be 52 in a few months. I'm wondering, "Am I losing my hearing a little bit? Should I get it checked?" So I understand a little bit of what you might have hinted at. What would you tell me?

P: Well, I think that I had to start listening to people around me because I caught myself a lot of times saying, "Huh? What? I didn't quite hear that," and it's incredible the advances that they've made in hearing aids. I mean my hearing aid, I can like go to conferences and things like that. I can take and switch it so it drowns out in the background noises. So I can actually hear people clearly around me. They were great with really taking the time to find out what works for me from a technological standpoint, and what I would be willing to use as well.

JM: What would you say to somebody who is wondering if they needed to get their hearing checked?

P: I know when I went in, they had – I think it was a free assessment. I'm not sure what it is now, if that's the same or not. But just going in and getting a comprehensive evaluation. It's completely different than getting like a hearing aid test somewhere else. I mean they have really high tech capabilities there and really do a really thorough evaluation. You can see everything. They show you where your weaknesses are. So it's pretty interesting just to see if you have problems.

JM: Patty, thank you so much for taking the time to share your story with us today.

P: Oh, you bet and one other thing I just have to say. I mean literally from the moment you call them, everybody there is just really nice and friendly and accommodating and really good – if you have to do it, you know.

JM: They want to take care of you is what you're saying, right?

P: Yeah, exactly. They were great. Just really nice people.

JM: Oh, that's wonderful. Well, thank you again.

P: You bet.

JM: Well, doctor, two for two.

DSM: All right! I like that.

JM: You mentioned the best way to get in touch. What's the web address again for your practice?

DSM: So it's the same as our name, www.SouthBayHearing.com.

JM: OK.

DSM: And that will have links so that you could order materials. It will have our phone number on it, so that you can call directly if you would like to book an appointment or need more information.

JM: What's the phone number just in case?

DSM: It's 310-375-6161.

JM: Oh, that's pretty easy to remember, 310-375-6161. That's great. Oh, we've got another phone call coming in. Let's go ahead and take that. Hi. Welcome to the program. Who's calling please?

P: This is Steve Facer.

JM: Hi Steve. How are you today?

P: I'm great, thanks.

JM: Good. Are you a patient of Dr. McBride's?

P: Yes. I've been a patient with Dr. McBride for several years now.

JM: Excellent. What has your experience been like?

P: Well, initially, I was – I think I was in denial about having hearing loss. But I could hear everything except my wife, at least that's what she claimed. After prodding from my kids and my wife, I went to see Dr. McBride and I found out that I had a significant hearing loss at higher frequency levels. When I was driving, I would hear overwhelming road noise because I heard the deeper tones so much better and that's why in the car, I just couldn't hear my wife.

So after a really thorough exam, Dr. McBride showed me a lot of options that would be available to me. You know, different types of hearing aids and explain to me how the brain works and hearing and did some additional testing and confirmed that I had lost some brain function. She said, "You know, I think Steve that as you experience the hearing aids, your brain will start to adjust and be able to really interpret this new hearing."

So I ended up selecting a Lyric hearing aid which is inserted in the ear canal and I – having never worn hearing aids before, I don't know how to really compare it to anything else. But it seems to me to be about as close to natural hearing as I could hope for. So the first thing I noticed when I got my hearing aids is that I said to my wife, I said, "Those birds outside are going to drive me crazy. Are they always like that?"

So yeah, I heard birds chirping, all sorts of things I hadn't heard and I just couldn't be any happier or any more happy than I am. I mean the service has been wonderful and my life quality is radically improved with hearing aids.

JM: That's great. Now, what would you say to somebody who might be in denial or hesitating?

P: I think get in there. Get it checked out. It has had a very positive impact on not only just personal relationships but it really has had a profound impact in my work life. I'm still actively working and so I found that there was an awful lot of meetings that I was missing that I now hear and so my effectiveness is really a lot higher and I would say that you don't put it off.

I don't know whether it's age-related or just environmental or whatever. But great hearing is an enormous asset that I was missing out on.

JM: That sounds great and thank you very much for taking time to share your thoughts with us today. I'm so happy for you and that this has all worked out well for you.

P: Oh, you're welcome. I appreciate the opportunity. I think the world of South Bay Hearing. Dr. McBride has been really helpful. Life has been great since I got my hearing aids.

JM: Have you suggested anyone go see Dr. McBride?

P: Yeah, I have a number of people that I work with. I travel a lot for business. So I encounter a lot of people from all over the country and of course they're not able to go to Dr. McBride. But I referred numerous people. In fact, I've suggested to one colleague of mine that he fly out from Atlanta and get his exam here and he could always get serviced by someone back there. So yeah, I would definitely advocate for Dr. McBride.

JM: Well, that's wonderful. Well, thank you so much.

P: You're welcome. Happy to do it.

JM: Well, doctor, as they say in hockey, hat trick! Three for three.

DSM: OK.

JM: That's cool.

DSM: People are great.

JM: It's obvious that they care about you and they do so because your care for them obviously comes through as well. So congratulations on that.

DSM: Thank you.

JM: That's great.

DSM: It has been a great business. I love what I do every day. I think people that work here understand we kind of have a higher mission in life. We are really about helping people live more abundant lives and it's really a good feeling to be able to affect people on such a personal level.

JM: Well, that comes across just obviously in our conversation today and also hearing from your patients and clients. It's great and congratulations!

DSM: Thank you. So when you're in the neighborhood, stop by. We will take a look in your ear.

JM: Sounds good to me and the web address again is …

DSM: www.SouthBayHearing.com

JM: All right. Well doctor, thank you so much for spending some time with us today. I mean this has been a fantastic conversation. I've learned so much.

DSM: Thank you, John.

JM: Yeah. No, this has been great. I've learned so much and I really want to thank you for taking the time to share your knowledge with us.

DSM: All right. Take care.

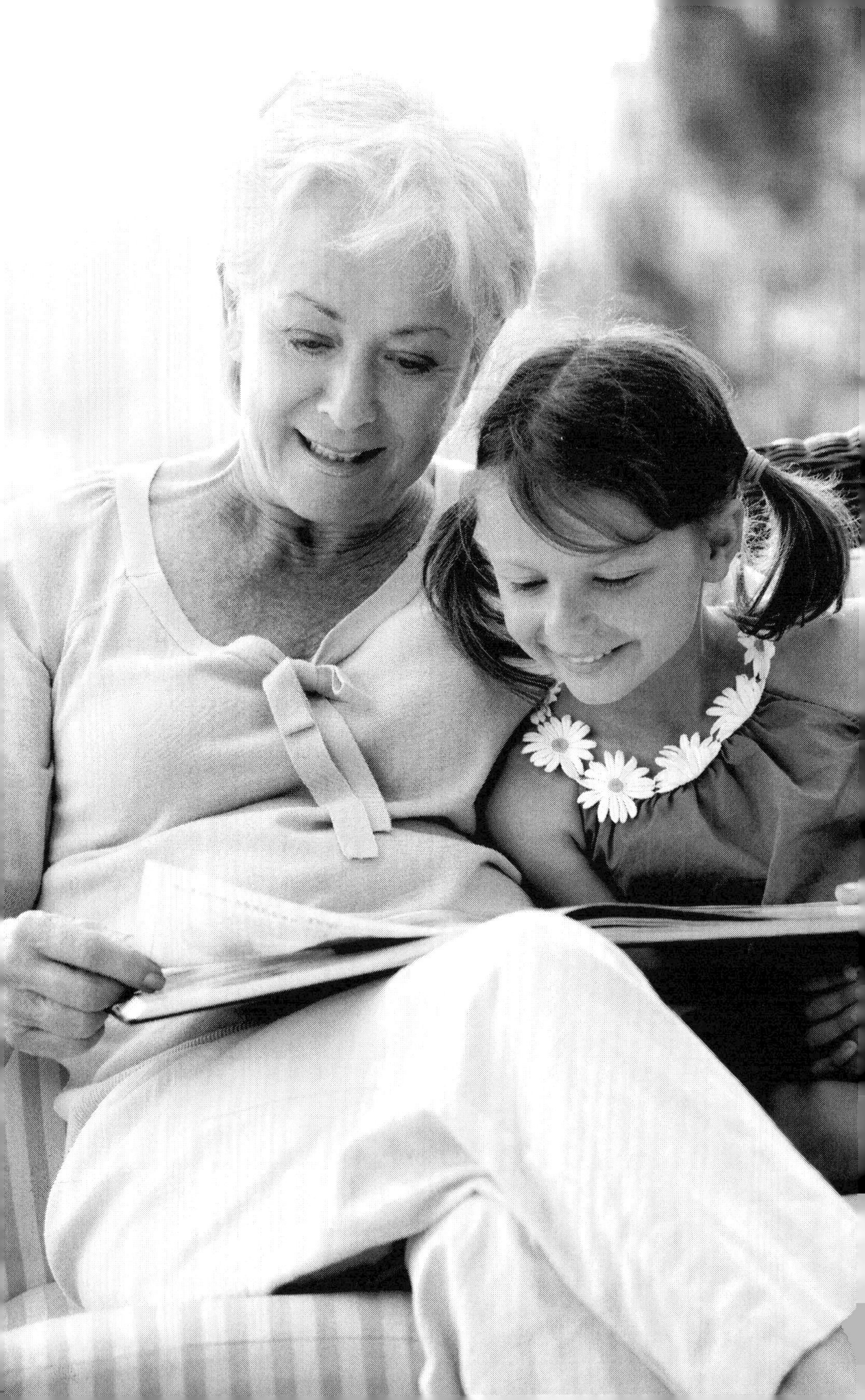

PREFACE

TODAY, APPROXIMATELY 48 MILLION PEOPLE in the United States are suffering from hearing loss. Yet, nearly 40 million of them go without treatment. Hence, the reason I wrote this book.

- *Do you want to remain independent and live an active life as you age?*
- *Did you know that hearing problems, even at the mildest stage, can lead to social isolation and increase the risk of dementia?*
- *Do you or a loved one have impaired hearing?*

Hi, I'm Dr. Keith N. Darrow, Ph.D. CCC-A, a trained Neuroscientist and practicing Clinical Audiologist. If you or a loved one has answered yes to any of the above questions, I encourage you to read this book and learn how you can live a better, more active, more engaged, and healthier life as you age. For over twenty years, I have been helping my patients, and their loved ones, break free of their hearing loss and live an active, engaged life—free of the worry, stress, and medical consequences of untreated hearing loss.

Hearing is what connects us to others. Hearing is a requirement for every personal and professional relationship we have; it is the building block of communication.

Hearing is also one of the major senses; in fact, I believe it is the single most important sense we have. While hearing certainly plays a major role in our fight or flight, prey vs. predator, and history as human beings, hearing today has the important role of keeping us communicating and connected with the world around us—at home, at work, and in our community. To further support my claim that hearing is the single most important sense we have, I offer the fact that the organ of hearing, the cochlea (AKA the inner ear), is embedded deep in the hardest bone in the entire human body, the petrous portion of the temporal bone (i.e. petrous means "stone/rock")—thus providing our organ of hearing significant protection.

I have put together this book to help you understand the dire consequences of untreated hearing loss and to introduce you to how today's medical options for treating hearing loss can not only help improve hearing, but also improve cognitive function, decrease your risk of developing dementia, depression, and falling, while also increasing your physical activity, and helping you live a happier and healthier lifestyle as you actively age.

Hearing loss has been listed by the Department of Health and Human Services as the third most common chronic health condition affecting seniors. ***Third!*** Hearing loss is estimated to affect nearly 50% of adults between the age of sixty to seventy years young, nearly 2/3 of adults between seventy to eighty years young, and the numbers only go up from there! As we live longer and science continues to increase life expectancy, we need to be best prepared to deal with this debilitating disorder and understand how it can impact our lives.

My journey up to this point has been filled with over twenty years of experience—from student to clinician to scientist to college professor and back to clinician and patient advocate. I was lucky to discover what I love to do in life, and as a result I have the good fortune to work with patients and their families every day as they embark on the journey of improved hearing and clarity.

While my elementary and high school performance wasn't much to speak of (in fact, I was dismissed from high school twice—but that is a story for a different day!), once I found my path of helping people understand and improve the process of communication in their daily lives, it all became incredibly easy for me.

In fact, I was on the Dean's List nearly every semester in college, graduated in the top 5% of my Clinical Audiology Program in New

York City, and went on to be the only practicing audiologist to complete a Doctoral Degree in the Neuroscience track at M.I.T. and Harvard Medical School.

As a trained Neuroscientist, expert in Speech and Hearing Bioscience and Technology, and a practicing clinical audiologist, I have a unique perspective on how the brain works and how hearing relates to overall health, well-being, and cognitive function. I also understand how treating hearing loss ***early*** (even before it becomes a problem that you and everybody around you can notice) significantly impacts your overall health and cognitive function and how it may significantly reduce your risk of developing dementia.

I believe that I am blessed to have the capability of transforming lives and families every single day. Treating hearing loss is not magic—it is the perfect mix of science and experience, which allows myself and my team to use advances in medical treatment of hearing loss, NeuroTechnology™, to stimulate the brain, improve cognitive function and mental health, and help adults remain independent. And the best part—it is simple for patients to manage and it's affordable!

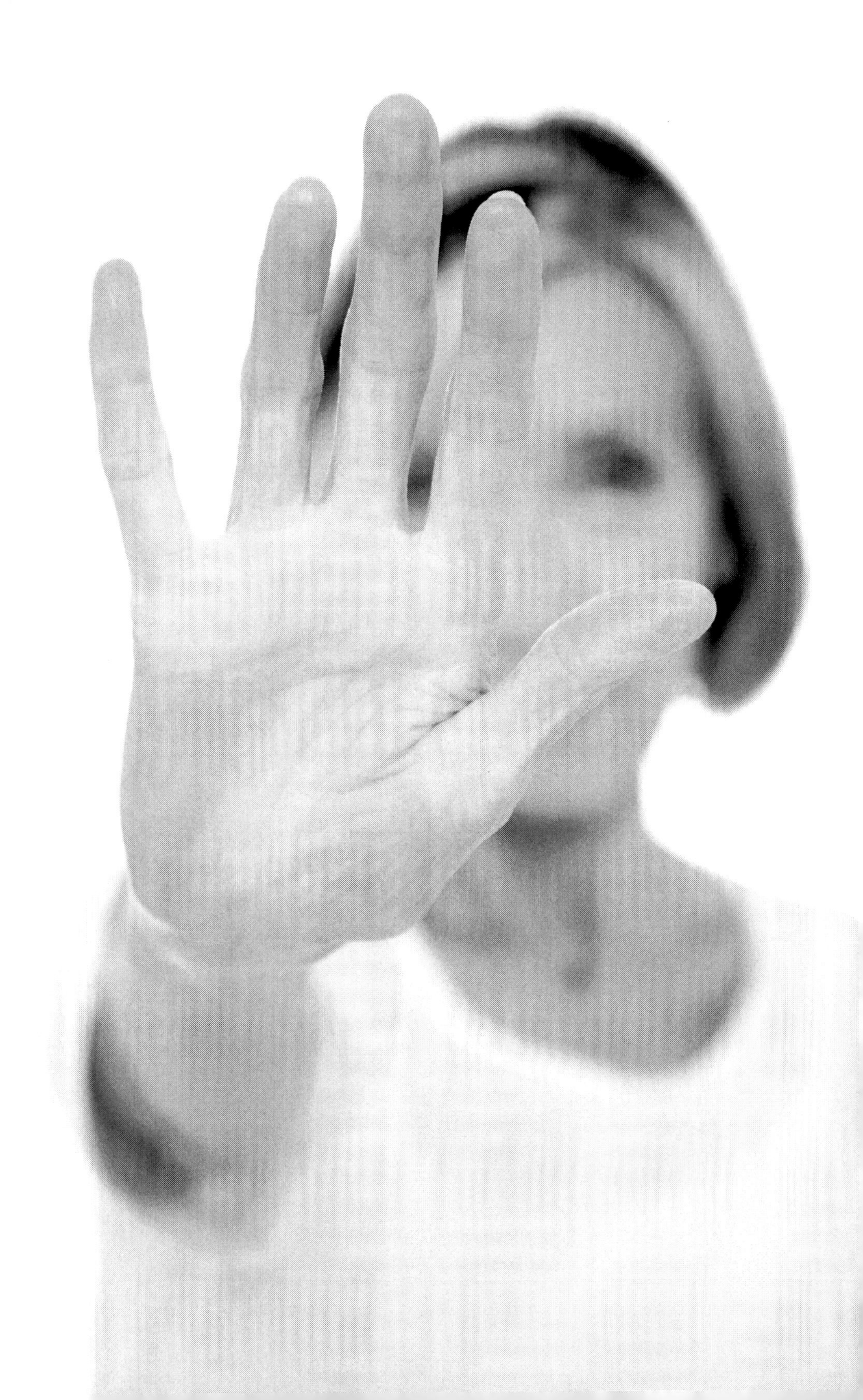

INTRODUCTION

The Top 5 Reasons People Avoid Seeing a Hearing Care Specialist

MY NAME IS DR. KEITH N. DARROW, and I'm a trained Neuroscientist and Clinical Audiologist! When people hear what I do for a living, they almost automatically…wince! They try not to be too obvious about it. (Hey, I have feelings, too!). It's okay; I'm used to it. The fact is, the less you know about audiology and treating hearing loss, the more reason you have to be afraid of it. Once upon a time, audiology meant one thing: big, heavy, ugly "beige bananas" to be worn on your ear to make sounds louder.

They were hard to put on, hard to make adjustments to, and, frankly, they were pretty terrible at doing anything other than making all sounds louder…this includes speech, background noise, loud ventilation machines, dogs barking, plates clanging, etc.!

For the majority of patients, wearing an old fashioned hearing aid meant avoiding certain social situations, restaurants, family gatherings, playing with grandchildren, etc. Many people still cling to the unfounded notion that all hearing aids are created equal and perform the same way they did back in 1982!

The fact of the matter is that audiology and the clinical science of treating hearing loss is more than just hearing aids. How much more? ***Audiology and the medical treatment of hearing loss is devoted to restoring an individual's clarity, restoring personal independence, improving cognitive function and mental health, and addressing the cognitive aspects of hearing loss that can increase the risk of developing dementia.*** Maintaining proper hearing and cognitive health has a significant impact on an individual's life—including all of his or her family, friends, and community members. Properly stimulating cognitive function and maintaining connections from the ear to the brain goes a long way in keeping a patient mentally competent, helping the patient remain autonomous, and helping keep at bay the mind-robbing diseases associated with cognitive decline (i.e. Alzheimer's). Treating hearing loss is a wonderful investment with life-long returns, and yet people still fear walking into a hearing health care provider's office for one simple reason—fear of the unknown!

Hey—it's okay to be worried about the unknown. We all have our reasons for avoiding the doctor. For example, I underwent aggressive management of atypical moles on my body (to avoid potentially pre-cancerous melanoma). I was scared. I avoided starting the treatment for several years. Until I realized that enough is enough…and I had my family bugging me to do something before it was too late. Starting treatment was the right thing to do, and while it was impossible to know the results had I not started treatment…the potential is there for me not having ever had the opportunity to write this book (if you catch my drift!).

For many, visiting a Doctor of Audiology is accompanied by many fears and anxieties. And for each patient, the experience is personal. There are reasons that patients typically wait seven years before being seen by a Doctor of Audiology and beginning treatment of their hearing loss. This list, *Top 5 Reasons People Avoid Seeing a Hearing Care Specialist,* has the most common conversations I have had with patients over the past twenty years about what took them so long to come in to my office.

While you may not place treating potentially pre-cancerous moles and treating hearing loss on the same level of importance, I promise that by the time you are done with this book you will understand why that premise is absolutely wrong and how the consequences of untreated hearing loss can negatively impact every part of your life, even rendering you dependent on others and at a significantly increased risk of developing dementia.

REASON #1 – The Patient Already Knows the Diagnosis Before He or She Ever Steps Foot in the Door.

Individuals with hearing loss have a tendency to wait nearly seven years before raising their hand and admitting they have a problem. Or perhaps it takes a family member nearly seven years to push his or her loved one through our office door! Either way, seven seems to be the "unlucky" number—I say "unlucky" because chances are very high that by the seventh year of experiencing the symptoms of hearing loss, significant damage has been done to the auditory system, which can lower treatment outcomes. I try to explain to all of my patients that hearing loss is a progressive degenerative disorder with neurologic involvement which undoubtedly requires early intervention. In lay terms, that simply means that your hearing will continue to degrade as you age, and the key to maintaining clarity and a higher level of hearing function (i.e. hearing in noisy environments) is to "*catch it early and treat it early.*"

I have empathy for the new patient who comes to my office to get his or her first hearing evaluation since grade school because I know, as does the patient, what the results will likely be. It is very brave for a patient to knowingly enter a medical office with the understanding that he or she is likely to receive the diagnosis of progressive degenerative age-related hearing loss. And that this disorder is neither reversible, nor is there a cure. However, there are restorative treatments available that can help the patient stay connected at home, at work, and in the community, and that can help stimulate the brain, improve cognitive function, and even reduce the risk of developing dementia (more on the connections of hearing loss and dementia later in the book!).

REASON #2 – The Patient is Not Sure of His or Her Insurance Coverage for the Procedures and Treatments Involved with Hearing Loss.

Regardless of when you read this book and which administration is running our country, insurance is a complex world to attempt to meddle through, and when it comes to hearing health care coverage, it can be even more murky. BUT…nearly every insurance company I have come across allows for coverage of one hearing evaluation per year by a trained hearing health care specialist (and more testing can be covered if medically necessary, i.e. if the patient notices a significant sudden change in hearing). A hearing evaluation is often considered "preventative" and, in many cases, does not require a referral from your physician.

While it is nearly impossible to speak for every patient and every insurance plan, this is intended to help ease the stress of navigating the process of hearing health care coverage. In fact, I believe any reputable hearing health care practice will have a deep understanding of the insurance regulations in its area and will be able to readily answer any questions you may have about your insurance coverage—or at least be willing to help you find the answer.

In my twenty years of experience in the hearing health care field, I have watched first hand as patient benefits for treatment of hearing loss have evolved—fortunately, in a direction that benefits the patient. Yes, medical treatment of your hearing loss may have an out-of-pocket cost associated with it, but I have seen insurance cover anywhere from 10% to 100% of the costs. And even if you were in the position of having 0% insurance coverage, treating hearing loss can be affordable—and you will learn throughout this book that treating hearing loss is truly priceless and can hardly be assigned a monetary value.

REASON #3 — Patients are Afraid of Being Sold Something.

It's like magic—once you turn the respectful age of sixty, you notice that the content of your mailbox seems to change. Nearly every week, perhaps a few times a week, you are "blessed" (I'm being sarcastic!) to have a full mailbox (both your physical and electronic mailbox) with literature about "essential vitamins for seniors," "how to choose the right assisted living residence," "how to invest your retirement money," "join AARP," and "which digital technology widget is best for your hearing loss." Somewhere along the line, hearing health care started down the dangerous road of becoming a retail transaction. Heck, I've even seen some hearing widgets sold at big-box retailers and chain pharmacies... although I don't know who would ever consider buying medical treatment for a progressive degenerative disorder alongside a giant vat of peanut butter! Like I ask my patients: "*Would you get your colonoscopy performed at one of the big-box chains? NO...so why would you treat your hearing loss there*?" I don't blame the patient for sometimes entering the office thinking he/she is going to be "sold" something.

My best advice is to steer clear of anybody trying to sell you something. If we go back to Reason #1 above, the patient is likely already nervous because he or she knows the medical diagnosis before ever even stepping foot in the office. Combine that with the fear of "being sold something" and that makes for a pretty nervous patient with his or her guard up.

Unfortunately, much of modern medicine is turning into a commercial advertisement seen on TV that marginalizes the process of treating a medical disorder; and hearing health care is not immune to this. In my office, and the Excellence in Audiology member-clinics across the country, our belief is in the medical evaluation and treatment of hearing loss.

I believe strongly that the proper medical treatment of hearing loss is best left to the clinicians specially trained to understand, diagnose, and treat your hearing loss.

REASON #4 – The Cost.

Actual Cost

We all know somebody, perhaps a family member or a friend, who has spent a significant amount of money on a hearing aid gizmo only to use it as a paperweight or to leave it in his or her sock drawer. And the reason is because the glorified over-priced amplifier that he or she purchased was never truly designed to improve hearing or clarity—it was designed to just make sounds louder. This truly angers me, and while I do believe that the patient plays a significant role in his or her health care decisions and follow-up care, the health care provider also must have a significant responsibility to the patient—even after the patient has left the office.

I have heard many horror stories about patients spending upwards of $10,000 on a pair of hearing aid gizmos—YIKES! More often than not, this very high retail transaction very likely took place in one of the chain hearing aid sales shops (i.e. the "Miracle Hearing" and "Bellstone" shops. FYI the real names of these retail establishments have been altered in an attempt to reduce my chances of being sued!). And, sadly, all the patient got in return for his or her money was a hearing aid amplifier capable of making things louder.

When a practice and the providers are committed to the medical treatment of hearing loss, you can trust that you are in good hands. I believe that a hearing specialist must meet the strict standards required of Excellence in Audiology member-clinics and follow the medical model of treating hearing loss.

I have always believed that the patient needs options to help him or her invest in proper hearing health care. A reputable audiology practice understands that for some people, the upfront investment in hearing healthcare can be prohibitive. Patients must be provided with options. All Excellence in Audiology member-clinics will offer reputable creditors/banks to help establish a payment plan (some with 0% interest for up to 18 months, or even a longer-term payment plan with fixed interest rates). Recently I established an affordable subscription plan at my offices, called Treatment4Life™, which provides individuals with the opportunity to pay a one-time down payment and a small monthly fee thereafter with the advantage of full warranty (loss, damage, and repair coverage for life), complete access to supplies, batteries and service appointments for life, and no-cost automatic upgrades in NeuroTechnology™ for life.

Hidden Cost

What about the cost of ***not*** treating hearing loss? While research has yet to make the definitive finding that hearing loss can *cause* dementia (causality is often difficult in clinical science), the evidence that the relationship exists is overwhelming. Even more important is the mounting evidence that treating hearing loss may significantly reduce the risk of developing dementia.

Every day, 10,000 people turn sixty-five years young. This trend is expected to continue for at least the next fifteen years. And it is almost a guarantee that over the next fifteen years, science will continue to reduce the mortality rate and increase the average life expectancy. As a result, our health care system will be pushed to its capacity to deal with diseases such as cancer, diabetes, cardiovascular disease, etc. Perhaps the most prevalent, most costly, and most disabling of all diseases we will see sharply rise over the ensuing decades is dementia—the mind-robbing mental disease that interrupts and interferes with every aspect of life. Dementia is ***not*** a normal part of aging.

Every three to four seconds, another patient is diagnosed with dementia. Rates of dementia are estimated to triple in the next thirty years. Unlike the other diseases listed above, a physical body with dementia is estimated to outlive the individual's mental capabilities by ten or more years! It is estimated that the average cost, per family, to manage the medical treatment and care of a loved one with dementia can exceed $57,000 per year.

There is no cure for this catastrophic disease, but there are treatments available, including several ways to decrease your risk of developing dementia. **In fact, a study published in The Lancet journal indicated that the treatment of hearing loss as the single most effective means of preventing dementia.**

I encourage you to read my report detailing "9 Key Lifestyle Tips to Reduce the Risk of Developing Dementia." This report can be found at ***www.ExcellenceInAudiology.org.***

REASON #5 — Everybody *HATES* Hearing Aids.

Let's be honest. Everybody hates hearing aids. In fact, when you make a reference to old-fashioned volume-enhancing hearing aids, I think you could go so far as to say "Some hearing aids suck!" There you have it—I said it! I've been working with hearing-impaired patients for nearly twenty years and although my patients love improved hearing, they hate their hearing aids. I don't see a reason to tip-toe around this subject or ignore the fact that patients generally do not like using hearing aids. Nobody wants a medical disorder that requires physically tethering a device to his or her body to treat the medical condition.

People who wear glasses do not actually *want* to wear glasses (although I do know some people who wear non-prescriptive glasses because they feel that they look "cool"). I remember growing up in a time where people who wore glasses were sometimes referred to as "four-eyes" or other derogatory terms—fortunately glasses are now commonplace for people of all ages. I know that in the next few years, I will likely begin to hold the restaurant menu farther and farther away from my face in a dimly lit restaurant and when that happens I will need to invest in the proper treatment of visual impairment—whether I want to wear glasses or not.

For some people, hearing aids carry the stigma of meaning "I'm old and ready to die." And nearly every day I see a patient try and talk him- or herself out of investing in hearing health care treatment because "eh, I won't be around much longer anyway." My response is always the same: if you live for three more days, three more months, three more years, or even thirty more years (which is not unreasonable to expect from my fifty-eight year young patients), isn't it worth wanting to hear and understand everything and everyone else in your life? I also point out to patients that they will appear to look much older if they continue to say "What?" or "Huh?" all the time or, perhaps even worse, start to isolate themselves from the conversation.

I get it, and I respect that patients don't want to use a hearing aid, whatever the reason may be. Any reputable hearing health care provider will realize this, also, and understand the difference between traditional hearing aids and advanced NeuroTechnology™. Features in NeuroTechnology™ are specifically designed to treat the medical condition of hearing loss, improve cognitive function, and improve overall quality of life. As an added benefit, NeuroTechnology™ is incredibly discrete and comes in several invisible styles (more on invisible hearing-loss treatment options later in the book).

PART 1

FINDING A HEARING HEALTH CARE SPECIALIST

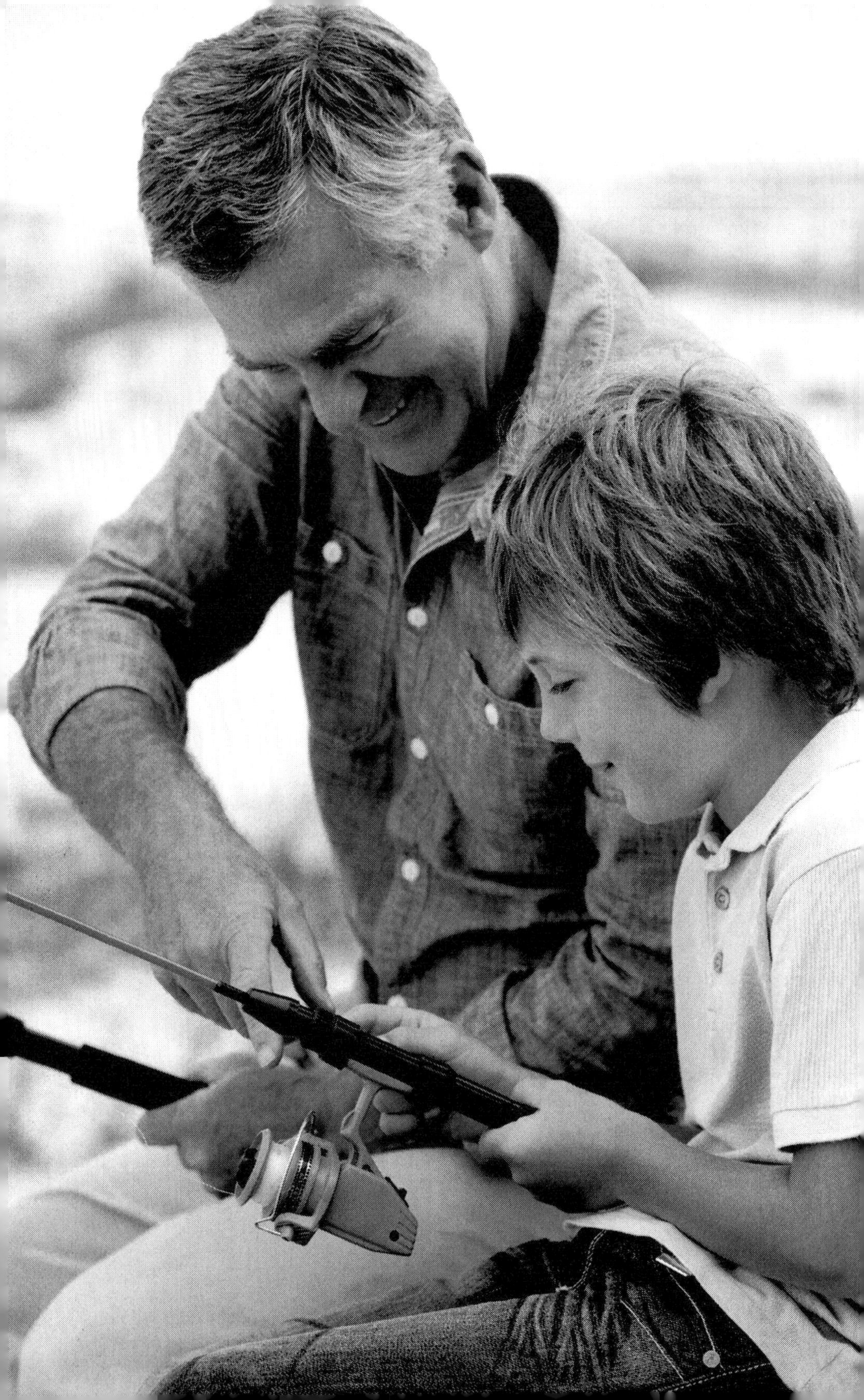

QUESTION #1

Why is hearing so important?

I believe most people can relate to my story: I watched my grandmother degrade as she crossed over from her seventies to her eighties. As she got older, her hearing got worse—and as the hearing got worse, her cognitive abilities declined. As a result, our ability to communicate with her was significantly strained. This is when I first knew that hearing loss must be correlated to cognitive decline (AKA dementia).

Communication is truly the basic building block of every relationship we have at work, at home with our loved ones, with our children, etc. Communication is a vital part of establishing and maintaining relationships. Watching my grandmother decline helped push me to be a better student, a better teacher, and a better clinician. When I decided to veer from clinical audiology for several years to focus on my studies at M.I.T. and Harvard Medical School, I decided to point my efforts at understanding the neuroscience of how we hear at the most basic level—from vibrating molecules of air to neural activity in the brain. Armed with this knowledge, I have been able to advance my patients' care to the highest level and help to set standards for testing and treatment protocol used in clinics across the country.

QUESTION #2

What are some of the early signs of hearing loss, and when should I see a hearing specialist?

Hearing loss is typically a slow, gradual onset disorder that silently (pardon the pun) affects the individual. The most common symptoms experienced by most (perhaps not all) patients are difficulty hearing in background noise, tinnitus, and thinking most people mumble or speak softly! Most people who experience the initial symptoms of hearing loss do not even realize it is happening. It is far easier to blame the acoustics of the room, the volume of the background noise, or the person speaking (i.e. "they mumble") than it is to accept that it's your hearing that is lacking. It is also difficult for many patients to rationalize the need for medical treatment of hearing loss because in some (ideal listening) situations (i.e. sitting at a table one-on-one in a perfectly quiet environment) may not be much of a challenge. But the truth is…

A Mild Hearing Loss is a Major Problem!

The first symptom of hearing loss for most patients is difficulty hearing in complex listening environments. If you take the time to reflect truly and deeply on your communication breakdown, I believe you will begin to recognize some of the initial symptoms of hearing loss. Are you having any difficulty when there are a few people at the kitchen table? Or when the kids come over? Or when communicating with your grandchildren? Or when you are at a social gathering (i.e. sharing a meal with friends and you can't seem to follow the conversation, yet all the other people seem to be enjoying themselves and following the conversation)? It is in these types of scenarios when hearing loss can really start to rear its ugly head and you realize that you are no longer an active part of the conversation. The result is a slow retraction from contributing to the conversation because you may feel embarrassed, and thus you continue to further isolate yourself and find yourself not truly engaging in conversations and relationships. And this is how even a mild hearing loss can really begin to impact your quality of life and relationships with others.

In addition to the importance of maintaining an active, engaged life with family and friends, early treatment of mild hearing loss is important for maintaining proper brain health. Simply put: Hearing Care is Health Care™. Your hearing drives your conception of everything and everybody around you; thus, hearing is essentially driving cognition at all times. It's driving memory. It's driving your image of the environment around you. You don't turn hearing on or off; you can't close your ears like you can close your eyes. There really isn't a sense or portion of your brain that isn't connected to your auditory system.

And I believe this speaks to how important hearing is to live and to thrive. We are bombarded with sound at all times and the brain is constantly, in real-time, making decisions as to whether or not certain sounds are important, trying to figure out how to categorize the sound and if it is important to store away and remember it for reference at a later date. A mild hearing loss can take away significant portions of the auditory world around you—and is likely the reason behind why patients with untreated hearing loss are at a significantly higher risk of experiencing a devastating fall.

The lack of cognitive stimulation that accompanies even a mild hearing loss is also associated with cognitive decline and dementia. Reports from Johns Hopkins Medical Center (and others) indicate that a mild hearing loss can increase the risk of developing dementia by 200% (up to a 500% increase for those with a severe hearing loss).

Like every major medical condition, the key to successful management of the disorder is early intervention. ***"Catch it early and treat it early!"***

QUESTION #3

Why, and how, should I choose a specialist for my hearing loss treatment?

I get this question so often that I developed a Top 10 List (although it's not nearly as fun as David Letterman's Top 10 Lists). This list can help a patient understand "why" they need to choose a specialist and "how" to choose the right specialist to trust with the treatment of their hearing loss. For a more detailed report than what is provided here, visit ***www.ExcellenceInAudiology.org*** for the full report.

The Top 10 Things You Must Know before Choosing Your Hearing Health Care Provider

❶ Is He or She a Specialist?

Hearing health care consists of both Audiologist and Hearing Instrument Specialist; both working towards the same goal—to help more people struggling with hearing loss. Audiologists are clinically trained hearing health care specialists that take on several extra years of training in order to provide the most thorough diagnostic evaluation and complete the most comprehensive treatment plans aimed at restoring hearing clarity. Hearing Instrument Specialist are trained and licensed professionals that dispense hearing aids. These hearing health care providers perform auditory rehabilitation, which is likely to include the use of NeuroTechnology™ that provides proper stimulation to the auditory system. This is a fancy way to describe how we normalize the way our brains process the incoming sounds in order to achieve maximum clarity, especially in background noise. While there are many hearing health care providers, less than 2% of all audiologists are Excellence in Audiology members.

As the leader of the Excellence In Audiology movement, I don't just treat hearing problems; I also teach clinicians across the country how to become better hearing health care providers. In fact, I have shared my knowledge and taught hundreds of hearing health care specialists throughout the world. By teaching and interacting with many clinicians, I am able to stay at the cutting edge with the best treatment options for my patients.

Another sign of a great specialist is he or she can show you a before and after of a similar case that he or she has previously helped. We know all ears are different, but with the 100,000+ ears our member-clinics have restored clarity to, we can show you a similar case to your specific hearing situation.

❷ Does the Hearing Health Care Provider Have a Medical Office (or a Sales Office)?

In the audiology world, it is not hard to open up shop on a shoe-string budget and call yourself a specialist. When you are searching for a provider, make sure you understand the clinician's credentials and medical affiliations. Often times, smaller offices with limited staff and audiology providers are somewhat limited in their service offerings and stability.

If you find a hearing care provider with the best credentials and an office that is inviting and in a medical setting, you have found a specialist who understands the importance of hearing health care and will be around for years to come to help you and your family best understand and address your hearing needs. For a list of Excellence In Audiology member-clinics, visit ***www.ExcellenceInAudiology.org.***

Excellence in Audiology member-clinics are located across the country with hearing health care clinicians of the highest caliber who insist on the best practice (often setting the standards for best practices) for their patients and loved ones.

❸ Does the Specialist Think Brain First?

Everybody thinks "we hear with our ears," and while that is partially correct, the process of hearing actually happens at the level of the brain. Today's hearing loss treatments are far more than a simple "amplifying" device behind your ear. The neuroscience behind modern treatments is focused on the brain, cognition, and the comorbidities of untreated hearing loss (comorbidity is defined as a disorder that co-occurs/is correlated to hearing loss). If your clinician thinks hearing first and *not* brain first in his or her treatment plan, you are missing out on many long-term lifestyle benefits. NeuroTechnology™ is aimed at restoring lost clarity, providing noise-canceling filters for noisy background situations, and soft-speech enhancers that emphasize the speech of those soft-speakers in your life.

When searching for your hearing health care provider, make sure you find a specialist that understands the significant negative impacts of untreated hearing loss on your brain. To find a local clinician who has been recognized for their commitment to thinking brain first in treatment plans, prescriptions, and protocols, you can visit the website ***www.ExcellenceInAudiology.org.***

❹ Do They Include a Free Consultation at the Initial Appointment?

Most audiologists and hearing specialists offer free consultations for new patients so that you and your family can get expert advice about treatment needs, options, and timing before making this important investment.

During your first evaluation and consultation, be sure your questions are being answered, your concerns are being addressed, and you are being educated about all of your treatment options. The clinician should include a comprehensive written report during, or after, the evaluation at no charge.

❺ Does the Specialist's Office Offer Guarantees? If So, What Are They?

No matter which hearing health care provider you choose, ultimately you are not making a small investment—in both time and finances. That being said, it is important to know that your clinician is going to stand behind his or her medical treatment plan. Every Excellence in Audiology member-clinic offers multiple guarantees.

In addition to a 100% Money-Back Clarity Guarantee, be sure your specialist offers a lifetime guarantee on service and prescription programming.

Rest assured—your hearing health care is my priority. Thus, I stand by everything I've recommended in this publication and why I have chosen to lead the Excellence in Audiology movement.

❻ Is He or She Using the Latest Technology and Treatment Options Available?

Audiology today differs a great deal from years past. Computer-designed NeuroTechnology™ devices and wireless technologies dramatically increase the precision with which we restore clarity and boost hearing ability. Scientific verification of device settings, while in your ear (referred to as Real Ear Measurements) maximize the precision of NeuroTechnology™ benefits. As an added incentive, today's NeuroTechnology™ are discrete and virtually undetectable to the user and others. In fact, a new category of NeuroTechnology™, known for being invisible, can offer the most discrete, cosmetically pleasing option placed deep in your ear canal to make the entire treatment a well-kept secret!

❼ Does Your Investment Include Treatment Supplies?

Each hearing care office has its own fee schedules, and specialists often charge differently for procedures. All specialists should offer you a contract which clearly spells out the investment for you or your loved one's treatment before it begins.

❽ Does the Specialist Charge for Follow-Up and Emergency Appointments?

Each time a patient embarks on the journey of improved hearing, there is an adaptation period for the user's ears and brain to adjust. This period can take thirty to forty-five days and is individual to each patient. In addition to the complex cognitive changes that happen when restoring hearing clarity, patients will notice significant improvement in some hearing situations and perhaps not as much in some other situations. This is common in the initial process of hearing loss treatments. I believe every patient is entitled to complimentary customizations for their NeuroTechnology™ prescription.

Keep in mind, if your NeuroTechnology™ is broken or damaged due to non-compliance with care, protection, and maintenance, this may result in repair charges. As a simple rule, if you do your best to avoid breaking your NeuroTechnology™ and follow the simple guidelines that your audiology specialist shares with you, then you should have no additional costs for customizations, even if it's an "emergency."

❾ Does the Clinician Make You Feel Special and Comfortable?

When you meet with your hearing health care provider, the person you are trusting with your hearing health care, you need to be in a comfortable and welcoming environment. Each Excellence in Audiology member-clinic I work with understands the importance of hearing and the distress that can be involved with making the decision to treat one's hearing loss. The entire experience from beginning to end, including a welcoming staff, should be designed to help alleviate a person's feeling of anxiety or grief.

We believe every patient is special and must be made to feel that way every time he or she comes to one of our offices in need of hearing health care.

⑩ Does the Specialist Have a Great Reputation?

With the internet today, it is extremely easy to pull up ratings and reviews from patients. Simply go to Google and search for audiology reviews and ratings within your town. At the time of this report, my practice in Worcester, Massachusetts, and our Intermountain Audiology clinics in the west, along with Excellence in Audiology member-clinics across the country have amassed thousands of five-star reviews on Google, Facebook, and HealthyHearing.com. No other network even comes close to this number of reviews. In fact, most of our offices have other providers in their area that have either no ratings or many poor ratings.

And don't be shy about asking for references—go directly to the source! You have the right to call any audiology office and ask for a list of references, including other patients and local physicians that have volunteered to help advise patients as they first enter the (sometimes overwhelming) world of hearing loss and to help patients understand rehabilitation experiences from the first-person perspective.

QUESTION #4

How early in life should I have my hearing evaluated?

The Simple Answer

If you are over fifty, you should have your hearing evaluated.

Detailed Answer

I have tried to stress the importance of early diagnosis and treatment of hearing loss throughout this book and to each of my patients.

The American Speech Language Hearing Association, the American Academy of Audiology, and the American Medical Association have all considered the recommendation of including "hearing evaluation/screening" between the ages of fifty to sixty years young. I often use the catch phrase "Ears and Rears" as my way of getting people to remember to have their hearing checked when they turn fifty (and of course, have a colon cancer screening too!).

Similar to going to your primary care physician every year, obtaining a baseline hearing test can help to better serve you and your clinician as a guide to the medical recommendation at current or future appointments. Obtaining a baseline evaluation and discovering that you have normal hearing never hurt anyone!

Regardless of age, if you are noticing any of the symptoms of hearing loss (e.g. difficulty hearing in noisy situations, difficulty hearing the TV compared to others), if your family is suggesting you get a hearing test, or if you have ringing in your ears (defined as tinnitus), then it is time to take the first step and have your hearing evaluated and discuss treatment options.

Unfortunately, waiting too long can significantly impact the expectations and outcome of treatment, and sadly every hearing health care clinician I know has a patient they have had to tell he or she waited too long and the benefits of treatment will be minimal.

PART 2
FIXING THE RIGHT THINGS AT THE RIGHT TIME

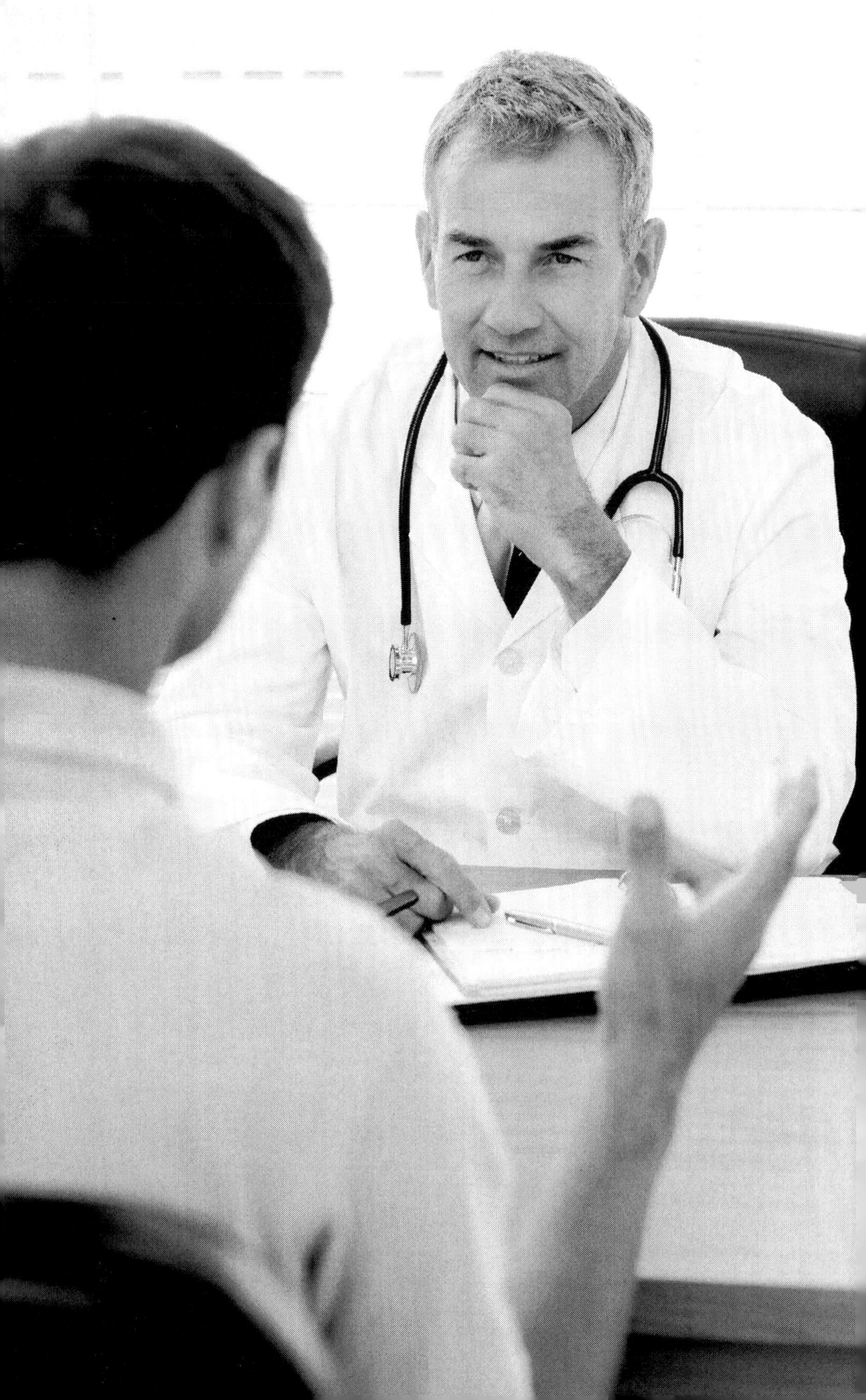

QUESTION #5

What will happen at the initial evaluation and consultation?

Every process has a beginning, middle, and end.

The Beginning

First things first…your specialist will ask you "Why are you here today?" (or some variation of that "why" question). This helps to set the stage for understanding your specific hearing related issues, concerns, and experiences. This conversation is the baseline to helping your specialist understand why you "raised your hand and are seeking help." While my job title may be "audiologist," this initial line of questioning is designed to help me better understand my patient at a deeper, more emotional level. I want to know my patient's experience with hearing loss and how it impacts his/her life. How does your hearing loss impact your relationship with your grandchildren? How does hearing loss impact your relationship with your spouse? Does hearing loss get in the way of your performance at work? Some of my patients wait their entire life to go fishing with their grandchild, and now their hearing loss is robbing them of the richness of that experience and getting in the way of developing a deeper relationship. As an audiologist, it is my job to treat ***your*** hearing loss and ***you*** as a person.

The Middle

Treating hearing loss is a process steeped in science, engineering, technology, and clinical medicine. There is also an "art" to treating hearing loss, and this skill is developed with years of experience. In order to develop the right treatment plan for each patient, first there must be the proper diagnostic procedures that test every aspect of hearing.

First your clinician will observe the ear canal to make sure the canals are free of any obstructing cerumen (ear wax). This is most often followed by a procedure called tympanometry that can rule out any medical condition causing hearing loss involving the eardrum and/or the space behind it, including the middle ear bones (the "Hammer, Anvil, and Stirrup").

The Beeps!

From there, it is important to establish the degree of hearing loss (ranked from mild to profound). Using the "raise your hand when you hear the beep" may conjure memories of having your hearing screened by the school nurse, but it still serves a purpose: establishing the degree of hearing loss. If your specialist stops testing you at that point and makes a recommendation for treating your hearing loss…I advise you to run as fast as you can! The information gathered from this test, although important, is only a piece of the puzzle.

The Words!

The most important testing we will perform is designed to assess your cognitive hearing, e.g. how well do you understand words in quiet and with background noise (after all, nobody comes to the office complaining that they can't hear beeps!). This line of testing will truly help your clinician understand how well you hear, and how well you process words and conversation.

Testing a patient's ability to hear words is often referred to as "Word Discrimination Scores/Ability." First the patient is asked to repeat a list of words at a near-normal conversational volume. Individuals with normal hearing will always correctly repeat between 96-100% of the words on this test. Individuals with hearing loss will not score nearly as well. For example, many people with a mild to moderate hearing age-related hearing loss will typically score between 50-60%—thus the patient is expected to miss 40-50% of what is said to him or her on a daily basis (especially when visual and contextual cues are removed and only hearing is utilized).

The next test is a repeat, almost exactly as just described, but performed a second time at a volume and clarity setting ideal for the specific patient's hearing loss. The result of this second round of word testing is referred to as the patient's "Hearing Potential Score." Most often the patient who formerly scored between 50-60% will now score 90% and greater; thus, treatment with NeuroTechnology™ is expected to improve the patient's hearing clarity to 90% and greater on a daily basis (especially in a quiet conversational setting). The patient is fully aware that he or she performed significantly better with enhanced clarity.

I mentioned earlier that the consequences of waiting too long to treat hearing loss can be dire. In some cases when the second round of word testing is completed, the patient's "Hearing Potential Score" will sometimes only be as high as 50-60%. In these cases, the outcomes and expectations for treatment are very dim (especially when compared with the patient who scored over 90%).

The Words In Background Noise!

The #1 complaint of every patient with hearing loss, and most often the first symptom of hearing loss, is difficulty understanding speech and conversation in background noise. Thus, it is critical that the clinician understands each patient's ability to decipher speech in background noise (again, without visual or contextual cues). This test, called the Quick Speech in Noise Test (QuickSIN™), is a means to quantify a patient's difficulty understanding and following speech in background noise.

Briefly, the sentence intended to be heard and repeated by the listener is presented at a clear and audible volume to the patient. With each new sentence introduced, the level of background noise (often referred to as "cocktail party noise") is increased in increments of five decibels. The final iteration of the test is when the speech and background "babble" are presented at the same volume—significantly taxing the auditory system and its noise-reduction filters.

Individuals with normal hearing are typically capable of hearing every word at each level, and even most of the words at the final, most competitive level. In contrast, individuals with even a mild hearing loss can struggle significantly on this test when the noise is ten decibels less than the intended speech. The test is scored on a Hearing Handicap Scale and can range from normal, to mild, to moderate, to severe Hearing Handicap. A majority of patients with a mild age-related hearing loss will often score in the mild to moderate hearing handicap range, confirming his or her reported difficulty following conversation in complex listening situations.

The End

Once all the testing is complete, it is the clinician's responsibility to review all test results with the patient and with his or her loved ones. These results are personal and can help a patient better understand the difficulty he or she is dealing with on a daily basis. Understanding the results can also be just as important for family and loved ones.

Although an individual with normal hearing can only imagine what it feels like to suffer from permanent hearing loss, gaining an understanding of the degree of hearing loss, Hearing Potential Ability, and Hearing Handicap scores can help the loved ones gain perspective on what the patient is going through and how much of a strain hearing loss can be.

These test results will determine the medical treatment plan and help initiate the journey towards improved hearing clarity and cognitive health.

QUESTION #6

What if I still have questions after the initial consultation?

The initial consultation can be overwhelming for some people and for their family members—and can sometimes stretch to sixty minutes or more. In these situations, it can be difficult to ask every question, to process everything that is being said, and to understand the enormity of the diagnosis of hearing loss. Every patient of mine has my e-mail, office phone number, and I've even gone so far as to include my cell phone number on my business card. I believe in an open discussion and dialogue and that many patients, and perhaps their family members, will have questions that come up even after the appointment is over.

I always invite and encourage patients to bring family and loved ones to their appointments. Bring a spouse, bring a child, bring a grandchild—it's okay because your hearing loss impacts every one of these people.

It is important that the patient and his or her loved ones understand exactly what is happening with the patient, exactly what the degree of hearing loss is, how the disorder can impact his or her life, how it can impact his or her cognitive function, and how it can impact his or her risk of developing dementia, which often leads to loss of independence and even institutionalization. At the initial consultation, there will also be a medical recommendation presented for how to treat the hearing loss. There is no one-size-fits-all treatment plan. NeuroTechnology™ offers a wide array of options that are often dictated by the test results and patients' needs.

QUESTION #7

When is the best time to treat my hearing loss?

A.S.A.P. Hearing loss is associated with increased rates of diabetes, heart disease, kidney disease, thyroid disease, falling, and the development of dementia.

The longer you wait, the more you are depriving the brain of proper auditory stimulation, often referred to as *auditory deprivation.* Your brain is not getting the proper auditory stimulation and auditory cues that it needs to run at 100%. The brain is a very simple "Use it or Lose It" mechanism, and auditory input can help to provide the proper, constant stimulation our brains are accustomed to and designed to receive.

Hearing is not a sense to take for granted. Yet the statistics are alarming—it is estimated that only 20% of individuals with hearing loss actually seek medical treatment. Without the proper treatment of hearing loss, the brain is being asked to work on overload, constantly. I often use the analogy "living with untreated hearing loss is like asking your brain to drive sixty miles per hour in second gear."

In neuroscience, we call this "Cognitive Overload"—asking the brain to process auditory, visual, and other cues just to put together a simple sentence.

Consider this sentence:

> *Hi, Martha! How is your puppy doing? Is he eating and growing OK? I hope we can get our dogs together soon to play.*

If we filter this sentence through a typical mild age-related hearing loss with compromised clarity (e.g. difficulty with consonant discrimination), the sentence could be perceived as this:

> *i, Mara! ow i our uy oing? I e eaing and groing o? I oe e an ge our do ogeer oon o ay.*

I think you will agree that this is rather alarming. Remember earlier when we discussed patients with mild hearing loss missing 50-60% of words at near-normal conversational volume? This is what it could sound like to the patient with auditory-only cues. Of course, the brain will use visual cues, lip-reading, etc. to fill in the missing pieces—but the brain was not designed to take on that much stress and effort just to understand a simple sentence.

This cognitive overload is hypothesized to be one of the leading reasons that individuals with hearing loss can be ***FIVE TIMES*** more likely to develop dementia.

QUESTION #8

What if I am nervous about treating my hearing loss?

Undergoing treatment for any medical disorder can be overwhelming to patients and to their family members. Fortunately, today's Neuro-Technology™ has alleviated most of the worries and concerns about treating hearing loss. The technology is specifically designed to be discretely worn all day and fit comfortably in the patient's ear. With enhanced clarity features, background noise cancellation filters, and wireless connectivity, today's hearing loss treatment options are simple and sometimes even fun—you can connect your NeuroTechnology™ to all sorts of home electronics including light bulbs, coffee pots, door bells, etc.—but this is beyond the scope of this book!

QUESTION #9

Why can't we wait until next year to treat my hearing loss?

Hearing loss, for some reason, seems to be the perfect thing for patients to try and put off "until next year." Patients will try to rationalize their hearing loss: "Oh, this is normal for my age" or "Everybody mumbles." If patients don't understand the unintended consequences of waiting to treat hearing loss and the medical conditions associated with hearing loss, how can they be expected to understand the importance of starting treatment of hearing loss **today!**

Simply stated, the organ of hearing (i.e. the cochlea) has a finite amount of receptor cells—referred to as hair cells. The hair cells are akin to the rods and cones of the eye, which receive stimulation and pass along the information as a complex series of neurochemical signals to the brain. As we age, like most mammals roaming the planet, humans are genetically predetermined to suffer the effects of age-related hearing loss. This problem is becoming more prominent in our society as we live longer, more active and engaged lives.

With this progressive degenerative disorder, there is a gradual, continual loss of hair cells within the cochlea. These cells each have upwards of thirty nerve fibers responsible for relaying information to the brain to process sounds and conversation. As each cell dies with age and excessive exposure to noise (compounded by the combination of the two), the cells will die and so, too, will the attached neurons.

A recent study from Johns Hopkins found significant cerebral atrophy (AKA brain shrinkage) in the brains of individuals with hearing loss—likely the result of the progressive degenerative nature of hearing loss. The cerebral atrophy found in these individuals is reminiscent of the global cerebral atrophy observed in individuals with dementia.

Treating hearing loss early has many advantages—predicated on "Use It or (Continue to) Lose It." Treating hearing loss cannot prevent further damage caused by our genetics or prior exposure to loud noise, but it can help maintain clarity and fine resolution of speech understanding as the disorder progresses. For example, a study I worked on at Brooklyn College (CUNY) graduate school under the supervision of Dr. Shlomo Silman was attempting to understand the impact of only using one hearing aid when the patient had equal amounts of hearing loss in both ears. The results were pretty alarming.

The untreated ear's ability to perform word discrimination tasks significantly reduced compared to the treated ear. Looking back on these results, they almost seem like common sense—the brain was designed to receive input from two ears and can respond adversely if only stimulated by one. I often joke with my patients who ask, "Do I have to treat both ears?" by asking them "How many *Monopoly-men* do you know walking around with a monocle!" In all seriousness, the importance of treating hearing loss early cannot be understated. Maintaining the strength and vitality of neural connections of the ear to the brain is key to the successful treatment of hearing loss.

PART 3
FOCUSING ON A PLAN THAT WORKS FOR YOU

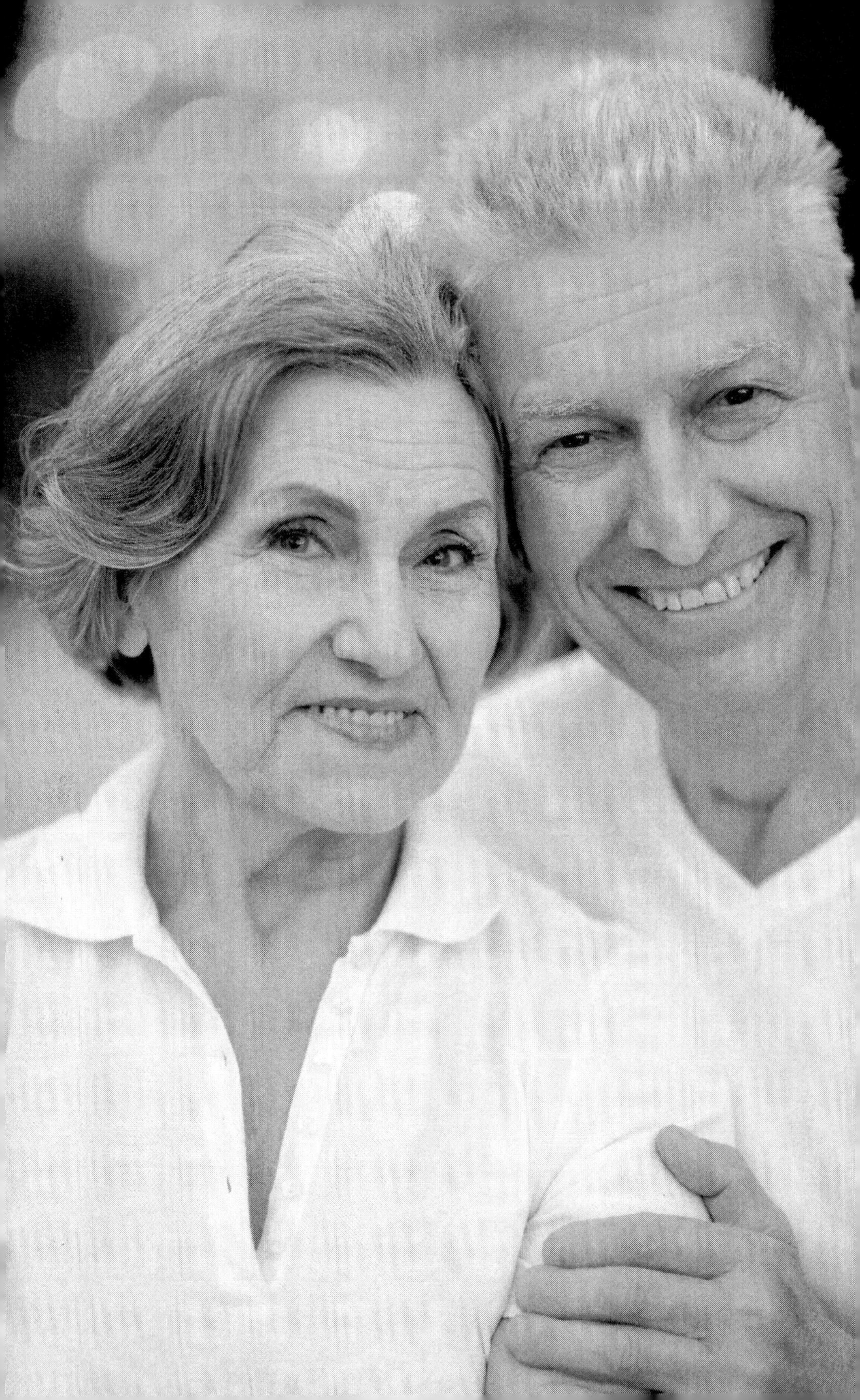

Is there an ideal patient?

The ideal patient is a person who understands both the medical and personal consequences of untreated hearing loss. A person who understands that his/her hearing loss is not just about him/her, but that hearing loss impacts his/her entire family, group of friends, and community. An ideal patient is somebody who is invested in his/her life, somebody who is invested in active aging, somebody who is invested in living independently, somebody who wants to stay engaged and who wants to be a part of the conversation, somebody who wants to be a part of his/her family and who wants to be a part of their community.

The ideal patient has to accept the cost-benefit ratio when it comes to treating hearing loss; and I hope that this book has helped patients understand that it's nearly impossible to put a dollar value on improved health. I believe the ideal patient truly wants to stay involved, wants to grow, wants to remain independent, and wants to make the most of every day and every relationship that he or she has. That is an ideal patient. If you are, or know someone that fits this description, please help them begin treatment of their hearing loss as soon as possible. You are always welcome at my center or at one of the Excellence in Audiology member-clinic in your area.

I suppose on the other side of the coin is the "not ideal patient"—the person who has his wife, his kids, and his grandkids basically pushing him into the office. That's not an ideal patient, although we have helped motivate many of them to realize what they need to do for themselves and their families. This type of patient must realize the severity of their situation and they must want to make a change. As you know, "you can lead a horse to water, but you can't make it drink."

QUESTION #10

What treatment options are available to me when I'm ready to start treating my hearing loss?

I get this question often as I travel the country meeting new patients, and even from family and friends. My answer is always the same: **NeuroTechnology™**. Advances in technology specifically designed to treat the cognitive aspects of hearing loss, not just make things louder, have significantly improved patient care and patient satisfaction.

But, my next response is always "*You must see an Excellence in Audiology member-clinic to determine which form of NeuroTechnology™ suits you and your hearing loss best.*"

While the most important factor in determining treatment is always based on the patient's hearing profile and health care history, specific options can be based on several factors including: addressing specific patient symptoms (difficulty in certain acoustic environments, tinnitus, etc.), dexterity (can the patient manipulate an invisible hearing device?), and personal preferences (color, size, etc.,). Your hearing health care provider can help you understand which form of Neurotechnology™, what shape and size, and which specific features can help you hear your best and keep you engaged in conversation.

QUESTION #11

What treatment options are available for the ringing in my ears (aka tinnitus)?

As a Neuroscientist and Clinical Audiologist, one of the most common questions, ***and complaints***, I get from my patients is about the 'ringing' in their ears! Tinnitus (pronounced either TIH·nih·tus or tuh·NYE·tus) is defined as a sensation of sound in your ears, sometimes in your head. Each person with tinnitus has a different sound experience; for most it is described as a "ringing" sound, but many patients also report a shooshing, buzzing, or wooshing sound—similar to the sounds inside a conch shell.

It is currently estimated that nearly 50,000,000 American adults live with tinnitus. Tinnitus is experienced by approximately 80% of people living with hearing loss.

Too many people dismiss the ringing, when in fact this sound essentially represents an internal alarm alerting you that something is not as it should be. Whether the tinnitus is constant, only noticeable in a quiet room or at night, pulsating or seems to have certain triggers (i.e. exercise or caffeine), it is important that the root cause of the problem be determined and a proper treatment plan be put in place with your hearing health care specialist. In some people, the tinnitus can interfere with daily life and result in depression, anxiety and affect concentration.

What is the cause of tinnitus?

The most common cause of tinnitus is damage to the sensory organ of hearing, the cochlea (i.e. the inner ear). The cochlea is to hearing what your eyes are to vision. Within the cochlea are tiny hair-like cells, called hair cells. When these cells are damaged, the nerves that connect the hair cells to the brain (and give us the ability to hear), become permanently damaged; and often times the ringing will ensue.

How Do the Sensory Cells In My Ear Get Damaged?

The sensory cells in the ear are most vulnerable to aging. Think about it—as we get older, we tend not to see as well or see as sharply as we used to, especially in low-light environments. Unfortunately, the same process happens in our ears as we age; we tend not to hear as clearly, especially in noisy situations.

Another common cause of tinnitus is excessive noise exposure, either a single intense noise (like a shotgun blast) or long-term exposure either from work or play (e.g. musicians, concert attendees, carpenters, machinist, landscapers, etc.).

But Why Do My Ears Ring?

Tinnitus is most often the result of a "Central Gain" in neural activity that occurs when there is a loss of proper neural stimulation from the ear to the brain. More simply, when the brain is not properly stimulated in individuals with hearing loss (even a mild hearing loss), the brain will increase activity to make up for the missing input.

This "Central Gain" is neurologically analogous to "Phantom Limb" phenomenon studied in neuroscience. In cases where damage occurs to the peripheral nervous system—such as when a solider loses a limb in battle—the central nervous system (aka the brain) will undergo adaptive changes that can often result in the perception of pain. Our ear's perception of pain is the ringing.

Treatment For Your Tinnitus

Unfortunately, too many patients have said to me, "I have tinnitus, and I've been told there is nothing that I can do about it." I emphatically say to each of these patients—that is not true! Is there a cure for tinnitus? No. Are there proven FDA-approved treatment options available to reduce, and in some cases, eliminate, the ringing? YES!

The single most effective treatment option available for patients suffering with tinnitus is NeuroTechnology™. The FDA (Food and Drug Administration) has approved treatment for individuals with tinnitus by providing the brain with restored proper stimulation. And while most people with tinnitus also suffer with hearing loss, that is not always the case. Fortunately, newly available NeuroTechnology™ has been designed for people with hearing loss and for individuals with (so called) "normal" hearing. Many studies show that patients who use the tinnitus support technology note a significant reduction in their daily tinnitus experience—with some even reporting that "the ringing is gone all day."

QUESTION #12

What if I have "total hearing loss" in one of my ears? (And what is a CROS System?)

As a general rule of thumb, hearing ability in the two ears should be near equal to each other. After all, your ears are the same age. If you have a history of noise exposure it was likely the same in both ears, and if you were prescribed a medicine with a side-effect that could impact hearing, it would impact both ears similarly.

But, in some patients, hearing in one ear will diverge from the other. This can result from a host of otologic issues, including viral infection of the ear, physical trauma to the ear, and of unknown origin (medically diagnosed as "idiopathic hearing loss," which is my favorite medical diagnosis because the root meaning of the phrase "idiopathic" is that the clinicians are idiots and don't know what happened! Ha! I don't say that to disparage any clinicians—it's just sometimes we can't figure out why the patient has worse hearing in one ear).

The separation of hearing levels between the two ears can sometimes be dramatic or even complete. Unfortunately, some patients have a "dead ear" (medically defined as anacusis) with normal hearing in the other ear. In other patients, there is an "asymmetric hearing loss" which implies hearing loss in one ear and even worse hearing in the other ear.

The brain was designed to hear with two ears, and it will function best with equal hearing in both ears. Binaural (two-ear) hearing has significant benefits that include increased sound localization ability (e.g. figuring out where sound is coming from in the room) and enhanced perception of speech in noisy situations. These characteristics of binaural hearing are often referred to as the "Binaural Advantage." If you know somebody with "lopsided" hearing loss, you will notice that she always strategizes to improve the listening environment by having the speaker(s) on her better hearing side.

While the course of treatment for individuals with significantly poorer hearing in one ear is different than the patient with symmetrical hearing loss, NeuroTechnology™ can be used to significantly enhance hearing and understanding in all listening situations.

Briefly, the most common NeuroTechnology™ used in these cases is referred to as a CROS System. CROS (Contralateral Routing of Signal) will take sound from the "dead" / worse side and route it over to the better side (even if there is some hearing loss in the "better" side). Using this technology allows the patient to access sound on the (otherwise) muted side of the body. While this patient may never perform as well as an individual treating equal levels of hearing loss in both ears, restoring perception of sound from the muted side of the body can offer significant relief in almost all listening situations.

QUESTION #13

Do they still make traditional hearing aids?

Yes, traditional hearing aids are still made. Mostly this traditional technology has been relabeled and is now masquerading as "new" over-the-counter (OTC) technology or personal sound amplification devices (PSAPs). Unfortunately, because the words "hearing aid" are very general and very common, it can be quite confusing for the patient. As I explain to my patients nearly every day:

"*Your father (or grandfather) wore traditional hearing aids (and he probably hated them). This older technology was intended to make sounds louder regardless of location in the room, regardless of the volume of the incoming sounds, and regardless of what the patient did or didn't actually want to hear.*"

As an audiologist seeing patients early on in my career, I was very disappointed by the limitations of the traditional hearing aid technology (and often embarrassed about having to relay the cost of the device—knowing the benefit would be limited, thereby limiting the patient's ability to remain socially engaged). This high level of patient dissatisfaction played a role in my decision to "take a break" from clinical audiology for nearly six years and pursue my studies in neuroscience.

QUESTION #14

So, what's the deal with new hearing aids and NeuroTechnology™?

(Most) new "hearing aids" are NeuroTechnology™.

To continue my answer from the last question: when I decided to come back to audiology as a clinical fellow at the Brigham and Women's Hospital in Boston and then as clinical professor at Northeastern University, I was instantly relieved at the giant leaps and bounds hearing aids had made towards improving listening experience for the patient (and thus increasing patient satisfaction). Around this time, the average patient satisfaction rating for traditional hearing aid experience was hovering around 70% to75% (as measured by the MarkeTrak survey).

If you now fast-forward another ten years to present time, the most recent MarkeTrack survey examining patient satisfaction with hearing loss treatment has shown an **improvement to 91%!** I believe this number speaks for itself.

Treatment of hearing loss with traditional hearing aids is (thankfully) beginning to be phased out and replaced with NeuroTechnology™ designed to enhance hearing in all listening situations, enhance clarity of speech details, automatically provide an increased boost of volume for soft speakers, stimulate the brain, and increase cognitive function.

QUESTION #15

What in the heck is an invisible hearing aid?

I saved my favorite treatment topic for last...*invisible hearing aids*. Like Wonder Woman's invisible jet plane—you can't see it, but it kicks butt! I get questions about this all the time from patients: "What is an invisible hearing aid?" and "Will my friends be able to see it?"

When treating hearing loss with NeuroTechnology™, I have two principles that I always follow:

1. Use the right Neurotechnology™ to treat the patient's hearing loss and improve cognitive health.
2. Respect the patient's desire for NeuroTechnology™ that is physically and aesthetically comfortable for them.

BUT... Principle #2 can *never* override Principle #1.

As a general rule of thumb in the tech world, the size of technology decreases over time. NeuroTechnology™ uses smaller, more powerful digital technology and processing to automatically adapt to the user's surroundings. I have always believed that treating hearing loss should require minimal effort from the patient. The hearing-impaired person needs to start using NeuroTechnology™ when he or she wakes up in the morning and then simply remove it before falling asleep—and do *nothing* in between! NeuroTechnology™ has ushered in the age of *effortless* hearing loss treatment.

Advances in design and technology allow for the user to be hands free—no more buttons for environment (i.e. push the button twice when in a noisy restaurant, push three times when in the gym, push the button four times when on the phone, etc.) and no more spin-wheels to adjust the volume up and down. Innovations in NeuroTechnology™ allow for automatic adaptation to dynamic environmental listening situations (e.g. listening to speech as you go from a quiet room to a noisy room), and it can automatically adapt to incoming volume to maintain the normal fluctuations in the volume of voices and background noise. The most advanced feature of NeuroTechnology™ is noise-cancellation that delivers increased access to clear speech in noisy listening situations (more on this in the bonus question!).

While NeuroTechnology™ is the circuitry inside the device, the device can come in different shapes and sizes to best fit your hearing loss and your ear.

NeuroTechnology™ Options for Treating Hearing Loss

Invisible Treatment Options

Once placed in your ear, this technology is hassle-free—you may even forget you're wearing the device! And that's the point. Hearing loss shouldn't hold you back, and neither should your hearing solution. Features in today's invisible technology options include:

- An invisible and custom fit
- A deep fit inside your ear canal and personal customization to you for all-day comfort
- Easy adaptation to new sounds with automatic volume control and adaptation to the listening environment
- Wireless streaming to your smartphone to keep you connected to your TV, music, and other media

- Sound comfort technology designed to provide distortion-free listening comfort for loud sounds while ensuring ultimate clarity

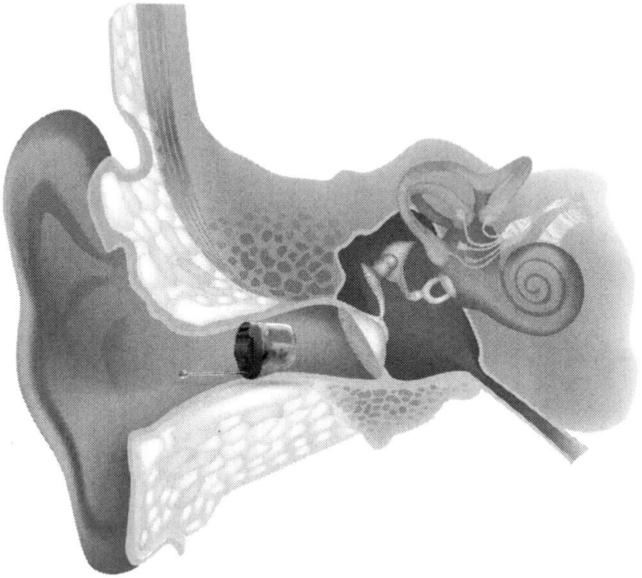

Invisible technology is seated comfortably in the ear canal for all day comfort and maximum discreteness.

Mini "Receiver in the Ear" Options

Groundbreaking NeuroTechnology™ is fast and precise enough to analyze and follow the dynamics of the entire auditory environment and differentiate between speech and background noise. Briefly (and without getting too lost in technical details), NeuroTechnology™ is capable of sampling sounds in the environment 100 times per second to make a decision on how to optimally perform and restore clarity; whereas traditional hearing aids were barely capable of analyzing the sound environment and capped out at a sampling rate of less that 5 times per second.

Advances in miniaturization of technology have led to the breakthrough of new NeuroTechnology™ found to support brain function, including working memory, selective attention, and processing speed (see Bibliography section for report from Dr. Desjardin, University of Texas, El Paso). These new devices have three features designed specifically to maintain the brain's innate ability to hear in all different listening situations:

- **Clear Hearing in Background Noise.** By separating important speech from background noise by as much as 10 decibels, this new technology provides 30% better speech understanding and clarity in noise*.
- **Enhanced Clarity = Enhanced Memory Recall.** Individuals with hearing loss can have difficulty with working memory, thought to be the result of distorted auditory input to the brain. NeuroTechnology™ can provide 20% more capacity to recall and remember words* by increasing the clarity of the signal being processed by the brain.
- **Reduced Mental Effort.** Many patients describe hearing loss as being "exhausting." Normal hearing is relatively effortless in most listening situations. But to an individual with hearing loss, even a simple conversation at work with a colleague or while out fishing with the grandchildren can require significant effort and use of all available mental resources, including lip-reading. Neurotechnology can offer the hearing-impaired user relief by reducing the "cognitive load" (e.g. mental effort) by 20%*; making the conversation significantly easier to follow in all situations.

**Compared to traditional hearing aids*

Other features include:

- Hands-free wireless surround sound hearing on the phone.
- Low-battery reminders. Devices can remind you by ear, phone, text, or email that your batteries (or your spouse's batteries) are low.
- Wireless compatibility with any TV to enhance the clarity of the signal.
- Control of your internet connected devices at home, including the thermostat, lights, and even certain cooking appliances.

Let's join in with all current NeuroTechnology™ users and celebrate!

Gone are the days of clunky "beige banana" hearing aids!

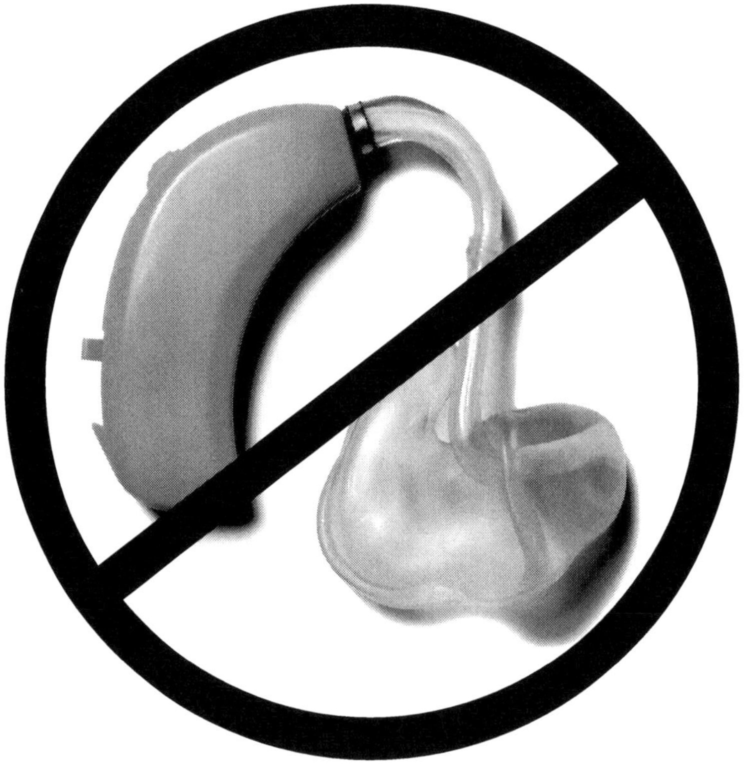

PART 4

FINANCING YOUR HEARING LOSS TREATMENT WITHOUT BREAKING THE BANK

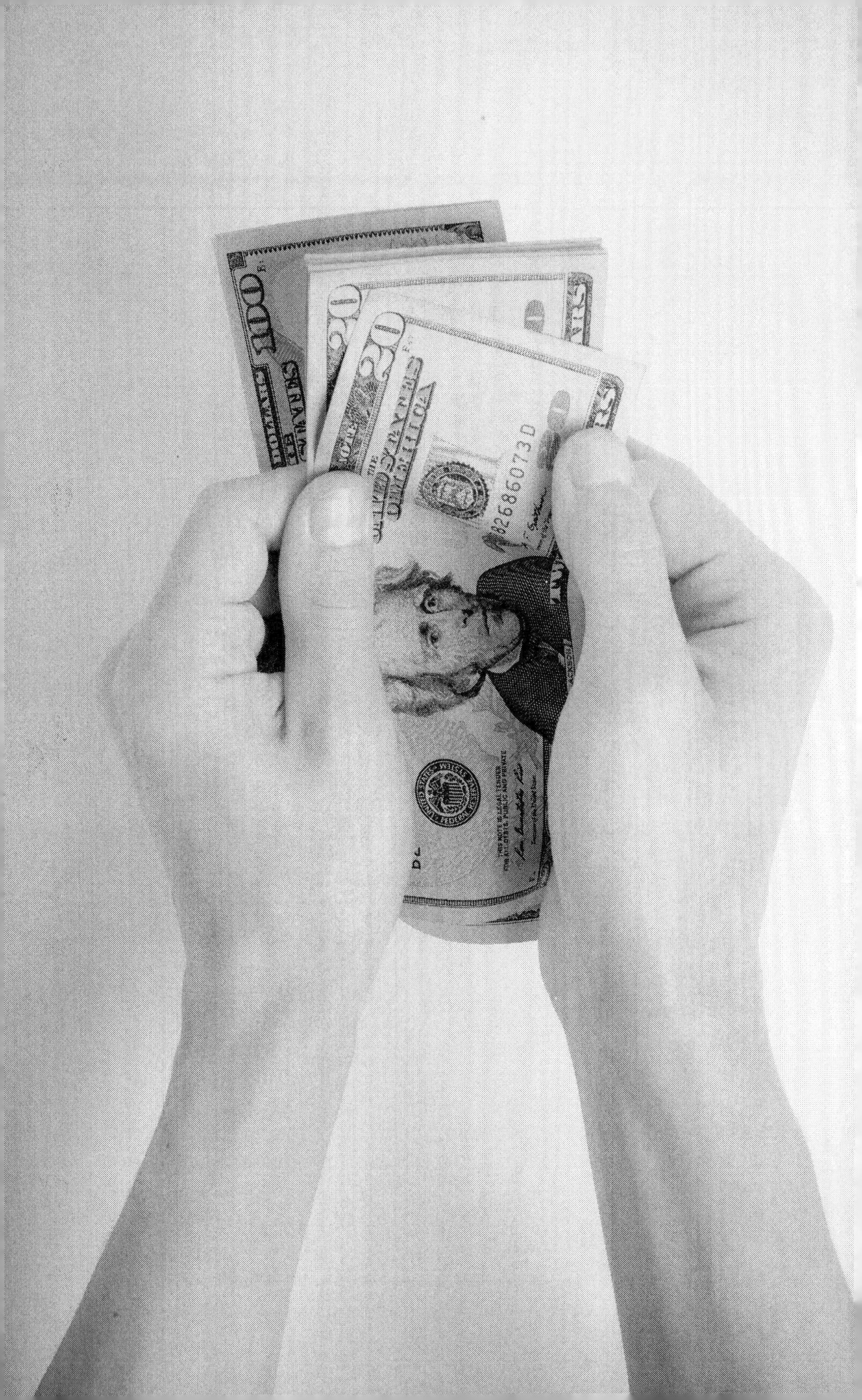

QUESTION #16

How much will my "new ears" cost me?

Answer: It depends.

Throughout this book I have alluded to NeuroTechnology™ treatment options as the "gold standard" of treating hearing loss. Specific recommendations will rely on a number of factors (e.g. degree of hearing loss, symptoms, amount of time living with untreated hearing loss, etc.). However, with that said, I have over twenty years of horror stories of patients trying to "*save a buck.*" I know patients who have thrown away $30, $300, even as much as $3,000 on a "sound machine in their ear" that amplifies volume. Some have tried traditional hearing aids that only make sounds louder; some have tried over-the-counter (OTC) devices; some have tried Personal Sound Amplifiers (PSAPs); some have even tried "mail-order" hearing aids. Regardless, each time the patient comes in professing his *mea culpa* and seeking forgiveness. I take no issue with patients trying to save money and make good economic decisions, but even with health care…you get what you pay for.

Treating the progressive degenerative nature of age-related hearing loss is no different than treating other major medical disorders as you age.

As an example, imagine yourself, or a loved one, in a situation where hip-replacement surgery is required. Could you imagine your surgeon asking the following question?

> *"Would you like me to replace your hip and restore 30%, 70%, or maximum percent mobility?"*

Here is another example, imagine saying to your heart surgeon, after he/she lets you know that you are required to undergo triple by-pass and heart valve replacement:

> *"Doc, if you don't mind, I'm going to shop on Amazon for a replacement valve to try and save a few bucks...even if it doesn't pump the adequate amount of blood to keep my body oxygenated and healthy."*

While both of these scenarios may seem far-fetched and ridiculous, unfortunately the retail aspect of hearing health care has "poisoned the well" for too many people living with hearing loss and has made treating hearing loss a very confusing, onerous process for the patient.

We trust all of our health care providers to use their knowledge and experience to provide us with the best, most medically sound treatment recommendation, ***regardless of price***. You should expect the same from your doctor of audiology. If your clinician is reputable (e.g. is referred to by local physicians, has many five-star reviews on Google, has readily available current patient liaisons to speak with, etc.), is an Excellence in Audiology member-clinic, and has longevity in the community, then you can rest assured that their pricing structure is standard and that the only variable is the cost of technology (pre-set by the technology manufacturer).

NeuroTechnology™ is the number one most effective, FDA (Food and Drug Administration) approved treatment for hearing loss and has the highest recorded level of patient satisfaction.

QUESTION #17

What is the cost of not treating my hearing loss?

Answer: Possibly a lot more than you think!

Throughout this book we have discussed the positive impact of treating hearing loss and the dire consequences of not treating hearing loss. It is difficult to assign a true monetary value to both of these scenarios, but I will give it my best shot!

Here are two examples.

1. **Hearing loss can increase the risk of developing dementia by 200-500%.** Treating hearing loss is reported as the single most effective modifiable factor to preventing dementia. Given these two medical research findings, it is not unreasonable to calculate the cost of treating a patient with dementia that could have possibly been avoided by treating his or her hearing loss at an earlier age. Statistics show that the average family will spend approximately $57,000 per year to cover health care costs and manage the care of a loved one with dementia.
2. **Hearing loss increases the risk of falls in seniors.** Treating hearing loss can significantly reduce the risk of falling. Again, given these two medical research findings, it is not unreasonable to calculate the cost of treating a patient who falls and compare it to the cost of treating hearing loss. Falling over the age of sixty-five is the #1 cause of injury related deaths. And once a person falls, he or she is two times more likely to fall again. The Center for Disease Control and Prevention (CDC) estimates that the average medical cost associated with a fall that results in hospitalization is over $30,000 (and the cost of treatment increases with age).

In addition to dementia and falls, co-morbidity of hearing loss (i.e. other diseases that are correlated with hearing loss) extends to diabetes, coronary disease, thyroid disease, and others.

QUESTION #18

How do I pay for my "new ears"?

Like any major medical procedure, audiology procedures can cost several thousand dollars, not all of which are covered by your insurance (depending on your plan!).

How much you will have to pay out of pocket depends on several factors, including the NeuroTechnology™ recommended, the procedures involved, and, of course, the specifics of your insurance policy. One way many of my patients pay for their treatment is by utilizing creative benefits. For example, using their Flexible Spending Account (FSA), financing at 0%, using tax returns, and even using the cost towards their medical expenses benefit on their tax returns (warning—I am not an accountant and do not even play one on TV—so always ask your accountant how to best proceed with all tax matters).

How to use Flexible Spending and eliminate the headache of using it!

Just to make sure we are all on the same page..."Flex Spending" is accessible through your work benefit package that allows you to set aside a certain amount of money per year, TAX-FREE, to be used towards medical expenses. **NeuroTechnology™ and treating hearing loss is a medical expense.**

Step 1—Sign Up Early!

Perhaps you already follow the "*5 P's to Success,*" (*Proper Planning Prevents Poor Performance!*) but in case you don't, this is one thing you want to plan early for so you can maximize the benefit. Many employees set higher limits than you think on the amount of Flexible Spending dollars you can contribute and access.

I have seen employees with as much as $2,500 and some with even $5,000 in Flex-Spending dollars available to them. Failure to sign up early could cost you more in out-of-pocket medical expenses, especially if your plan is not up and ready before you or a loved one needs to treat his or her hearing loss. If you have a new plan, work with your human resource contact to sign up early for next year in order to maximize your savings.

Step 2—Notify Your Employer of Family Status Change.

Different employers have different sign-up deadlines for the Flexible Spending plans, but typically at the beginning of the year your employer asks how much money you want to contribute for the year.

The problem with making annual decisions about health care coverage is obvious—life happens and sometimes it's nearly impossible to plan ahead that far! You may apply for a Family Status Change for changes such as marriage, birth, divorce, or loss of a spouse's insurance. These are opportunities to add more coverage for hearing loss treatment expenses.

Step 3—Choose Wisely!

Finally, give some thought to calculating how much money to contribute to your flexible plan at work this year and every year. If you are considering hearing loss treatment for you or a family member, visit the specialist's office for an initial consultation.

Your patient care coordinator(s) can help you plan exactly how much money you should contribute to help reduce your out-of-pocket costs when it is time to pay for and receive your NeuroTechnology™.

Step 4—Use It or Lose It.

Here's something you may not know (and frankly, has always puzzled me!): if you put more money in to your Flex Spending Account than you need or use, by law, you lose the money! Yikes!

BUT…you have three months after the end of the calendar year to submit claims for eligible medical expenses from the previous calendar year. Any money left in your account after this three-month period is forfeited.

To Finance or Not to Finance? 'Tis the Question!

As a human being with a family, home, and many other fiscal responsibilities, I understand the difference between things I ***need*** to buy and things I ***want*** to buy. Treating hearing loss is something that my patients ***need*** to invest in to ensure proper hearing and cognitive health. But not every patient is able to pay for treatment up front in a lump sum. A respectable hearing specialist will be able to offer their patients the opportunity to finance. I can't provide the details of every office, or every offer, but these are the common financing options I have come across:

- 0% interest for as long as twelve to eighteen months
- 12.9% interest with locked-in monthly payments for three to five years
- "In-house" financing plans with lower interest and even longer terms

What about the new "Subscription Model," Treatment4Life™, I keep hearing about?

Some Excellence in Audiology member-clinics are offering the new Treatment4Life™ option to their patients. I have always worked tirelessly to remove barriers for my patients to invest in proper hearing health care. I also recognize the dilemma current patients face when they have to upgrade from traditional hearing aids to NeuroTechnology™. This is why I have devised a plan for our Excellence in Audiology member-clinics to help more specialists help more patients.

With Treatment4Life™, patients are offered the option of an initial down payment with recurring (fixed) payments. This structure has several benefits that include:

- No-cost upgrade to new NeuroTechnology™ as future generations become available (approximately every three to four years)
- Complete warranty coverage that includes damage and loss coverage for the life of the NeuroTechnology™ program
- Free accessories for your NeuroTechnology™, including TV and telephone adapters
- Free service, free annual hearing evaluations, and free supplies (batteries, cleaning supplies)
- And more…

This is a fantastic resource for patients to be able to access premium level treatment plans with a fixed monthly cost…all with no worries about any future costs!

QUESTION #19

Does my insurance cover the cost of NeuroTechnology™?

This is a loaded question—and one that I can only answer in general terms because health insurance coverage is a complex ever-changing set of rules, regulations, and specifics that make it impossible to make a blanket statement regarding *your* coverage.

After twenty years of patient care and working with nearly every flavor of insurance coverage, these are my two take-away messages:

1. Nearly every insurance plan, including Medicare, will cover the cost of the comprehensive hearing evaluation.
2. Many patients have some coverage for the cost of treatment (e.g. NeuroTechnology™).

I acknowledge that "nearly every" and "many" are vague terms, but this is the world of insurance we currently live in. I have worked with patients that have $100 of coverage and some with $10,000 in coverage (not that it should ever cost you that much!).

TIP: Do not be afraid to pick up the phone and ask your insurance company point blank: **"Do you cover the cost of treating hearing loss?"** Also, don't be afraid to call back and ask again (you would be shocked how many times our office has called insurance companies seeking this answer only to get a different answer each time we call!). At my office, our Patient Care Coordinators will take the guess work out of the patient's hands and will work directly with the insurance company, and fight with them when needed, to maximize the patient's benefits and coverage.

BONUS SECTION

TREATING HEARING LOSS & YOUR OVERALL HEALTH

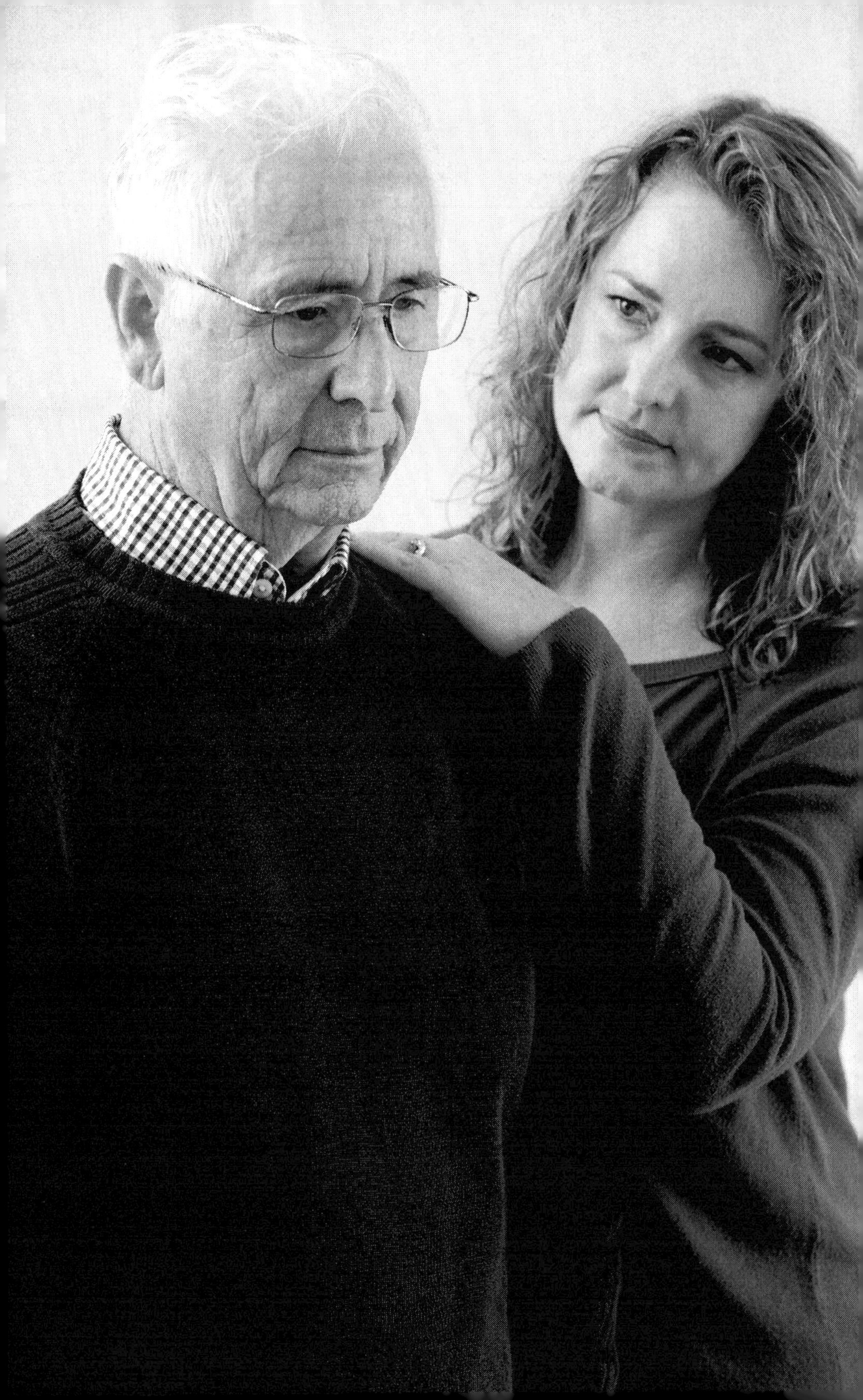

QUESTION #20

What is the research behind the relationship of hearing loss and dementia?

Age-Related Hearing Loss is a progressive and degenerative disorder resulting from the loss of receptor cells (i.e. the hair cells) in the ear. Consequently, there is a significant reduction of the quantity and quality of neural connections from the ear to the brain. This slow-onset disorder can have a significant impact on several key brain areas, including the memory, hearing, speech and language portions of cognitive function. Several key research studies have pointed to the potential links of hearing loss and dementia, including the groundbreaking work from Dr. Lin and his colleagues at Johns Hopkins Medical Center that indicate **hearing loss can increase the risk of Dementia by 200-500%.**

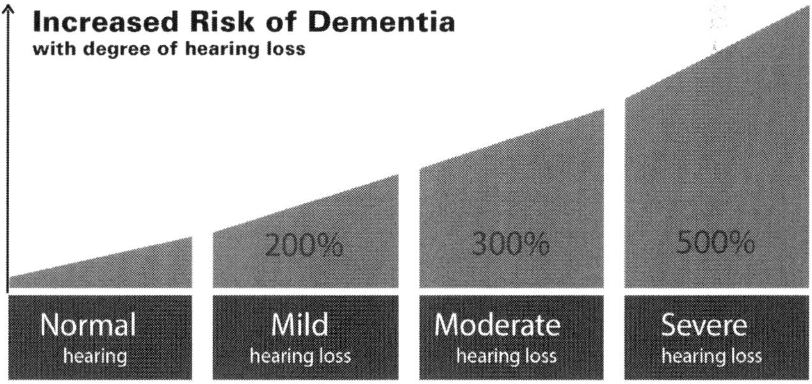

Summary data of relationship of hearing loss and increased risk of developing dementia.

The initial report first published in 2011 by scientists at Johns Hopkins Medical Center and the National Institute on Aging found that individuals with hearing loss (when compared to participants with normal hearing) are at a significantly higher risk of developing dementia as they age. The relationship of hearing loss and increased risk was rather simple: the more hearing loss they had, the higher the likelihood of developing the memory-robbing disease. "A lot of people ignore hearing loss because it's such a slow and insidious process as we age," Dr. Frank Lin (of Johns Hopkins Medical Center) says. "Even if people feel as if they are not affected, we're showing that it may well be a more serious problem."

Three risk factors associated with hearing loss and dementia include Social Isolation, Cerebral Atrophy and Cognitive Overload.

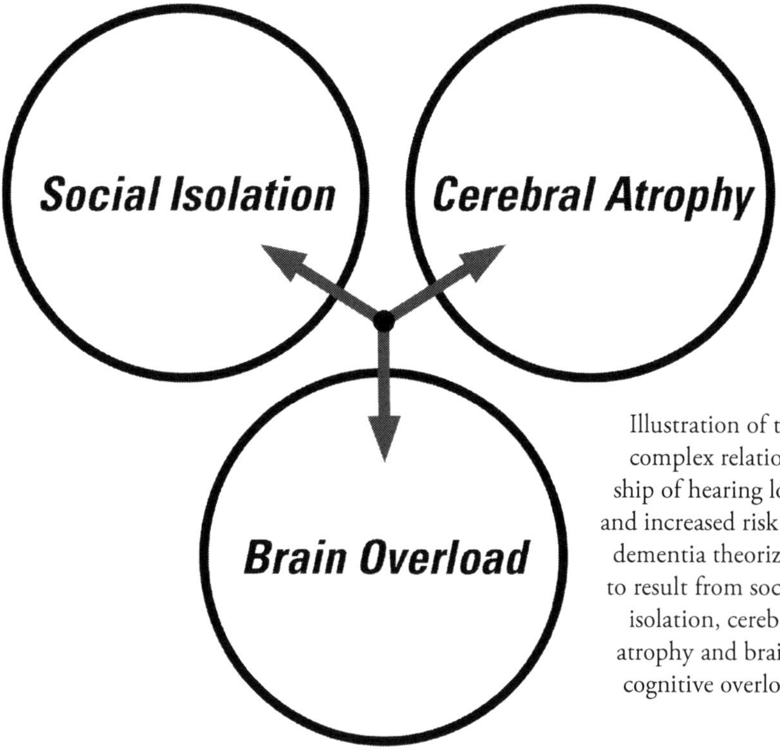

Illustration of the complex relationship of hearing loss and increased risk of dementia theorized to result from social isolation, cerebral atrophy and brain/cognitive overload

1. Social Isolation

The Impact of reduced social and physical activity. Withdrawal from social situations is common in individuals with hearing loss. Many studies cite feelings of embarrassment, fear of making mistakes in conversations, and feeling like you are not part of the conversation as the common rational for individuals with hearing impairment to separate themselves from family, friends and community. This retreat from social activity has even been found in individuals with a mild degree of hearing loss. In addition, individuals with hearing loss are less likely to engage in physical activity. Both increased social isolation and reduced physical activity are strong risk factors for the development of Dementia.

Blindness Separates You from Things,
Deafness Separates You from People.
— Helen Keller

Active Aging: How to Reduce Social Isolation

Active Aging—the process of optimizing opportunities for better health, continuing development of knowledge, and increased security in order to maximize quality of life as you age. The word "active" is used to describe a person's involvement with social, physical, economic, spiritual and civic affairs. We all share the same goal to maintain autonomy and independence as we age, and thus we must rely on preserving the tenants of interdependence (socialization and reliance on family and loved ones) and intergenerational solidarity (maintaining companionship with age matched peers) to insure active aging.

Both Social Isolation and Depression are risk factors for the development of dementia, and both increase as we age. Being a lifelong learner and staying active is important to maintain a healthy, active brain, and can also reduce your risk of cognitive decline and dementia. Some studies have shown that social activities, larger social networks, and a history of social contact are associated with better cognitive function and reduced risk for cognitive decline.

Tips for Active Aging include:

- Sharing a meal with family and friends 3–5 times per week
- Committing to an aerobics/exercise regiment
- Learning a new hobby each year
- Playing an instrument (or learning a new instrument)
- If you love to read…keep reading (and try to mix up the topics!)
- If you don't read much—try to read a book every other month
- Participating in classes at your local senior center
- Volunteering at a local hospital, shelter, etc.,
- Going back to school. Many local state Universities offer free tuition to people over 65!

2. Cerebral Atrophy (AKA Brain Shrinkage)

The association of a shrinking brain, resulting from the loss of neurons, with dementia has been long documented. Even people with MCI (Mild Cognitive Impairment) show signs up cerebral atrophy. In recent years, scientific studies using advanced brain imaging techniques (including fMRI - Functional Magnetic Resonance Imaging) have demonstrated that hearing impairment is associated with accelerated brain atrophy in both the overall brain, as well as even more advanced reductions in volume associated with the memory, hearing, speech and language portions of the brain.

Individuals with Hearing Loss can experience significant cerebral atrophy. The most significant reduction in cerebral volume occurs in areas involved in memory, hearing, speech and language.

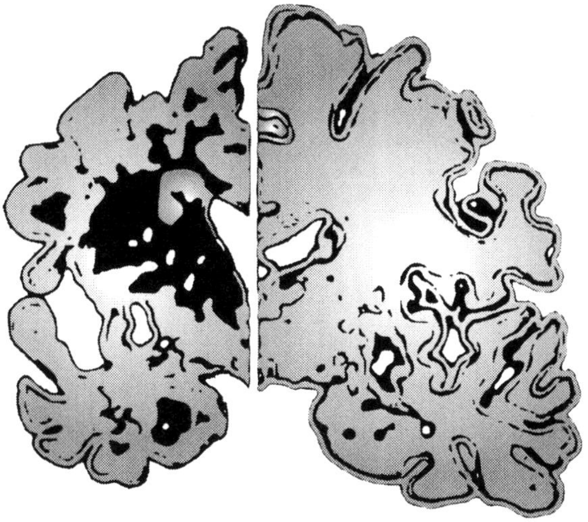

Brain With Hearing Loss **Brain With Normal Hearing**

Schematic representing the potential cerebral atrophy in an individual with age-related hearing loss.

3. Cognitive Overload (i.e. Working Your Brain Too Hard to Hear)

Hearing loss is not normal, and neither is the excessive strain that it can put on your brain. If you or somebody you love is experiencing hearing loss, you can observe this strain by watching the amount of effort required to follow a conversation. Patients will often joke and say "I need to put my glasses on so I can hear you better." Requiring these extra visual and lip-reading cues may seem a natural way to fill in the missing speech details, but long term these coping mechanisms may have harmful effects on cognitive function.

With hearing loss, the brain is constantly on "overload" trying to fill in the missing pieces, and follow the conversation. I often describe to my patients the taxing effect of hearing loss on brain function by describing the mental effort required to hear "is like driving 60 miles per hour in only second gear."

Increased cognitive load is considered a risk factor for developing dementia. Cognitive load, as measured by pupillometry (i.e. the size of the pupils indicates the amount of mental effort), can quantify how hard your brain is working to follow a conversation. Recent studies have found that individuals who treat their hearing loss do not work as hard to listen (i.e. have a reduced cognitive load) and have as much as a 20% increase in memory recall when following a conversation, even in noisy environments.

QUESTION #21

Can I reduce my increased risk of developing dementia by treating my hearing loss?

As I discuss the relationship of hearing loss and dementia with my patients, each seems to have the same follow up question for me: *"Doc, if I treat my hearing loss, can I prevent or reduce my risk of developing dementia?"*

Thankfully, the data appears to be trending towards a resounding "***Yes***!" Recent reports have found a significant positive impact of treating hearing loss on cognitive health.

Treating Hearing Loss and the Impact on Cognitive Function

In a recent study investigating the relationship of treating hearing loss and cognitive function, it was found that current hearing loss treatments can improve brain function in people with hearing loss. It is understood that hearing loss, if left untreated, can lead to emotional and social consequences, reduced job performance, and diminished quality of life. Recently, studies have even shown that untreated hearing loss can interfere with cognitive abilities because so much mental effort is diverted toward understanding speech (i.e. cognitive overload).

The research was aimed at measuring core cognitive functions in subjects in their 50's and 60's beginning hearing loss treatment for the first time. After only two weeks of treatment, cognitive testing began to reveal a significant increase in scores for recalling words in working memory and selective attention tests, and that the processing speed for which participants selected the correct response was significantly faster. In summary: after only a couple of weeks, participants exhibited significant improvement in their cognitive function.

Treating Hearing Loss and the Impact on Risk of Developing Dementia

Since 2011, multiple long-term studies have provided strong evidence that treating hearing loss may eliminate the increased risk of developing dementia. **Dr. Lalwani at Columbia University noted that treating hearing loss...**

> *may offer a simple, yet important, way to prevent or slow the development of dementia by keeping adults with hearing loss engaged in conversation and communication.*

Perhaps the most definitive report comes from the Lancet Commission, which presented a new life-course model documenting potentially modifiable risk factors for dementia. The Commission's report suggests that treating hearing loss is the **single most effective modifiable factor to preventing dementia.** Other modifiable factors include reducing depression, increasing physical activity and reducing social isolation – each of which is positively impacted by treating hearing loss.

QUESTION #22

Can I really expect to be more socially active and engaged once I start treating my hearing loss?

Yes. Throughout this book, I have been providing countless examples of how treating hearing loss can profoundly impact a patient's life and mental health. Frankly, connecting the dots of treating hearing loss to improvements in overall health and personal independence is simple.

If you ask your primary care physician "Doc, what do I need to do to be healthier?", the answer is guaranteed to include reduce stress, increase physical activity, stay socially active and engaged, lose weight, and eat healthy. Treating your hearing loss can help you achieve most of these goals. And achieving these goals is the key to healthy active aging.

There are countless medical studies that find that people who do not treat hearing loss suffer from increased rates of depression, decreased socialization, and decreased physical activity. As an example, the National Council on Aging reported that individuals who do *not* treat hearing loss suffer from depression, anxiety, and decreased social activity. In contrast, individuals who proactively treat their hearing loss find improvements in relationships with family members (spouse, children, grandchildren, etc.), increased self-esteem, and improvements in overall quality of life.

Connecting the Dots of Treating Hearing Loss and Improving Your Life

- Treating hearing loss can increase physical activity, reduce stress and anxiety, help with losing weight, and ultimately mean living a healthier and more independent lifestyle.
- Treating hearing loss can increase clarity of speech and the ability to follow conversation in background noise, increase socialization, help reduce the risk of depression, and ultimately mean living a healthier and more independent lifestyle.
- Treating hearing loss can increase auditory and environmental awareness, decrease the risk of falls, and ultimately mean living a healthier and more independent lifestyle.
- Treating hearing loss can increase cognitive function, can reduce the increased risk of developing dementia, and ultimately mean living a healthier and more independent lifestyle.

Hearing loss can be isolating for so many people for a multitude of reasons. **But it doesn't have to be.** If you've made it this far through the book, you have come to understand the importance of treating hearing loss and taking care of your brain—and how these two are connected.

I wish you luck and happiness as you embark on the journey of treating hearing loss, restoring clarity, increasing independence, and keeping a healthy and fit brain!

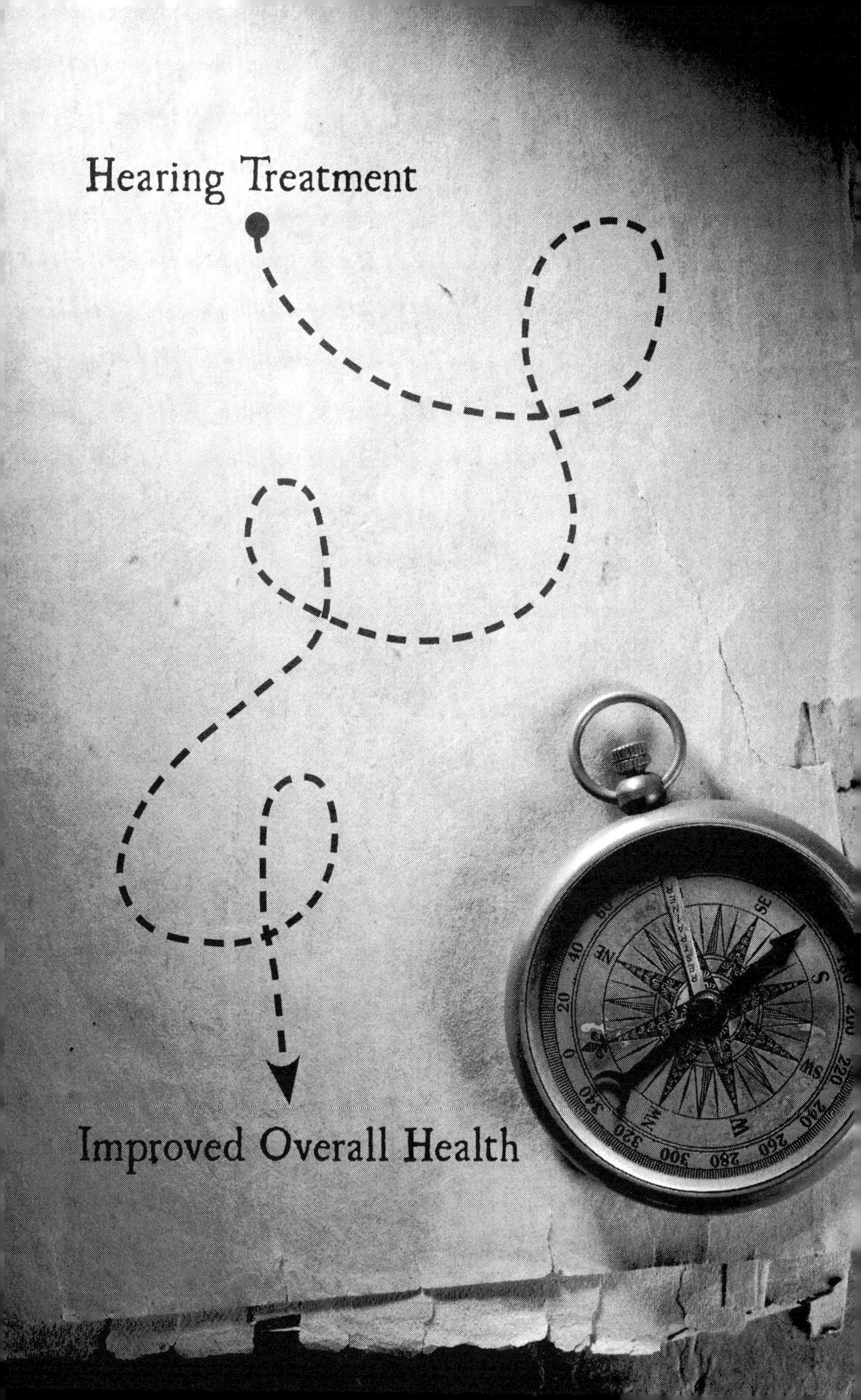
Hearing Treatment
Improved Overall Health

EPILOGUE

You Had Questions and I Hope I've Provided Answers

SO, THERE YOU HAVE IT! Twenty-two of my patients' most popular questions answered (for your convenience, I've included a handy FAQ directly after this epilogue that summarizes most, if not all, of the questions we've just covered. Consider it a handy "quick reference" of sorts).

The fact is no book can ever answer EVERY question for every patient. Every case is unique, just as every patient with hearing loss that I treat is different. What I've tried to do is provide you with the basics and, hopefully, the confidence you'll need to ask further questions of your own hearing care specialist when the time comes.

This is your hearing, your brain, and your overall health we are talking about here; never be afraid to insist on being heard and having your questions answered by your clinician. Now that you're armed with the answers for today's most frequently asked audiology questions, you can finally make the right decision for you or a loved one when embarking on the journey of medical treatment for hearing loss.

When you are ready to take the next step to improve your life, your cognitive function, and your hearing health, please call:

(310) 421-4396

to Schedule Your Treatment

South Bay Hearing

FAQS

A RESOURCE GUIDE OF FREQUENTLY ASKED QUESTIONS & TERMINOLOGY

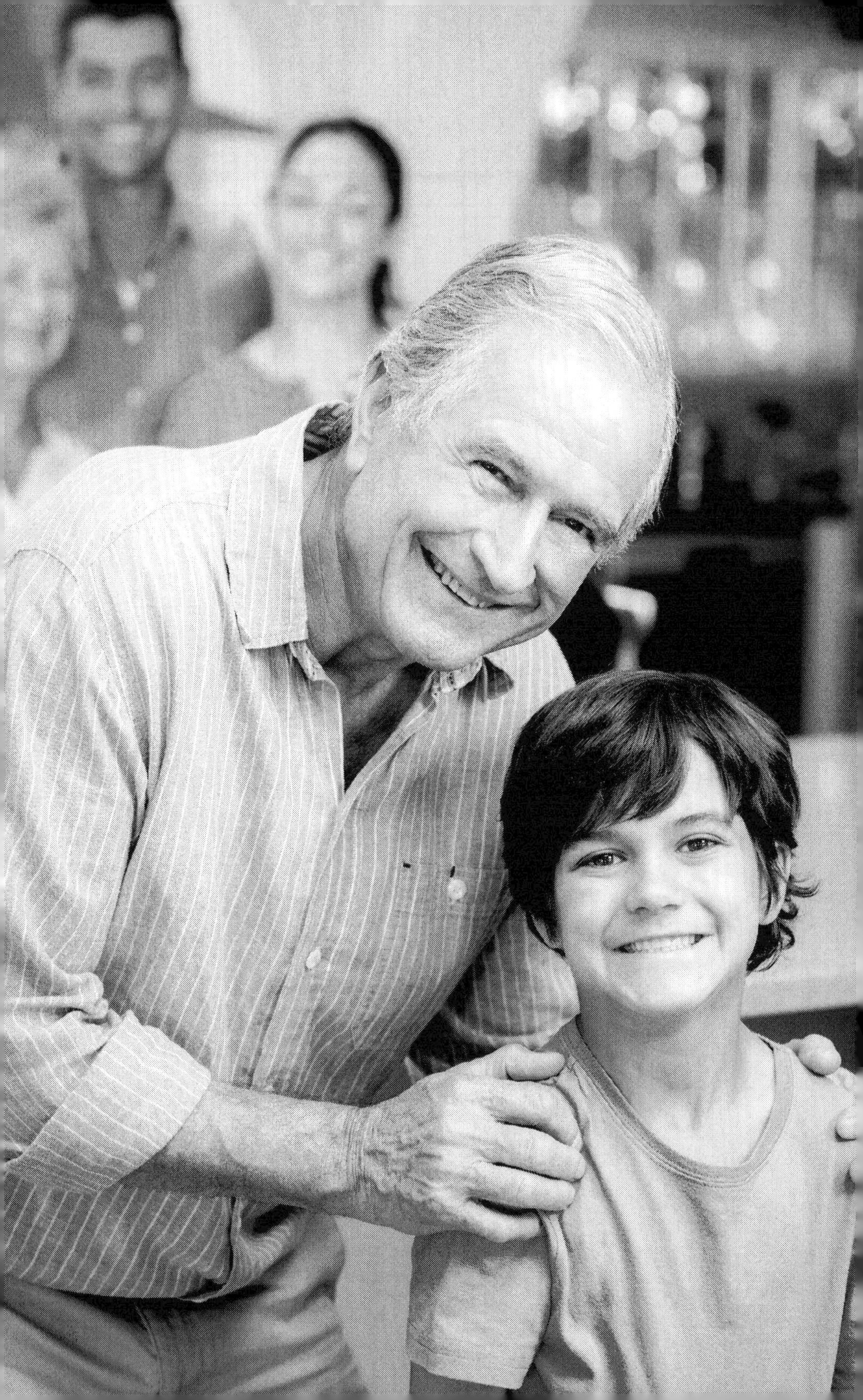

What might happen if I wait to treat my hearing loss?

Even mild hearing loss can be a major problem for a number of reasons. Hearing loss can increase the risk of developing dementia and is correlated with several other major diseases including diabetes, coronary disease, and kidney disease. Early treatment also improves the treatment prognosis and expected outcomes.

Who are some famous people who've invested in treating their hearing loss with technology?

The list is quite long! A (much) abbreviated list includes presidents Reagan, Clinton, and George H.W. Bush, and other celebrities and famous athletes including Huey Lewis, Lou Ferrigno, William Shatner, Pete Townshend, Whoopi Goldberg, Derrick Coleman, Congressman Jim Ryun, Phil Collins, and Brian Kerwin.

Will I be able to afford NeuroTechnology™?

Yes. Not only are hearing loss treatment options more affordable than ever, but insurance, payment plans, flexible spending accounts, the Treatment4Life™ program, and a variety of other financing options make this an all but moot point.

Will being fit with NeuroTechnology™ be painful or obvious to others?

No and no. Advances in miniaturization of technology have helped develop the most light-weight, discrete, and sometimes completely invisible technology ever used to treat hearing loss.

Will I have to miss work or other social activities once fit with NeuroTechnology™?

The initial comprehensive evaluation and treatment procedures will take between one to one and a half hours. Follow-up visits after that will only take between fifteen to thirty minutes. Patients walk out of the office after the first appointment and go about their lives...only now they can hear ***MUCH*** better!

Is it really such a big deal if I don't treat my hearing loss?

Yes. Too many people believe that their hearing loss is "normal for their age." There is no such thing as "normal" or "age-corrected" hearing loss. Hearing loss is a progressive degenerative disorder that will continue to negatively impact your life and cognition the longer it goes untreated.

What are some of the warning signs that I may have hearing loss?

Early symptoms of hearing loss include difficulty following conversation in background noise, experiencing tinnitus (ringing in the ears), having to turn up the TV louder than others need it, asking people to repeat often, finding yourself needing to read lips to hear better, difficulty understanding on the phone, and your family bugging you about getting help.

What kind of side-effects can result from NOT treating my hearing loss?

Untreated hearing loss is implicated in increased risk of falls, development of dementia, diabetes, coronary disease, depression, as well as increased stress and reduced physical activity.

Why should I choose a specialist to treat my hearing loss?

Hearing loss is a major medical condition and has been listed as the **third most common** medical disorder impacting seniors. Unfortunately, loopholes in many state and federal laws allow for traditional hearing aids to be sold in retail establishments, including some of the big-box discount stores. These traditional hearing aids are most often older models and are only designed to amplify sound.

NeuroTechnology™, designed to treat the cognitive aspects of hearing loss, is the "gold-standard" and considered "best practices" by audiologists and board-certified specialists in private practice audiology clinics.

How do I know if my hearing care provider is a Doctor of Audiology?

This is typically pretty easy to figure out by searching the internet or even calling the office. I've never been bothered by a patient calling to confirm my credentials prior to his or her arrival—in fact, I believe this shows a proper amount of due diligence on the part of the patient and a true investment in his or her hearing health care. Most states will also provide a list or search tool online to find licensed and certified providers.

What is a Patient Care Coordinator?

During your initial consultation(s), you will usually be assigned a patient contact person—we call this person a Patient Care Coordinator in our office—with whom to schedule appointments, confer with for rescheduling, and, of course, help you get answers to any and all questions you may have at any point in the process.

Why are follow-up visits important?

These are wonderful opportunities to ask questions you may have missed the first time, get further details from your specialist, and bring a family member to learn about your diagnosis and treatment plan.

Why is early treatment so important?

Since we recommend adults fifty and older to have a comprehensive hearing evaluation, we have coined the term "Ears and Rears"! This is meant to remind people to add hearing to their list of medical appointments once they turn fifty. At fifty, if the patient is found to have hearing loss, it is critical to start treatment early to avoid some of the devastating consequences of untreated hearing loss. Alternatively, if the patient has normal hearing, a baseline will be established and used for comparison at follow-up appointments.

What if I don't believe in early treatment of age-related hearing loss?

Unfortunately, for many patients it takes nearly seven years for them to admit they have hearing loss (or to succumb to pressure from family members) and start treatment. By this time, the hearing loss will typically be at a moderate degree or beyond and, in some cases, treatment outcomes can be negatively impacted. To assure a positive prognosis and improved treatment outcomes, hearing loss must be caught early and treated early to maintain positive connections to the brain. *"Catch it early and treat it early!"*

What is sensorineural hearing loss?

Sensorineural hearing loss (SNHL) is a hearing impairment that results from damage to, or dysfunction of, the inner ear (cochlear) and/or the auditory nervous system. Age-related hearing loss is a form of sensorineural hearing loss.

What is a conductive hearing loss?

Conductive hearing loss (CHL) is a hearing impairment that results from damage to, or dysfunction of, the outer ear (pinna and ear canal) and/or the middle ear (the eardrum or ossicles—hammer, anvil and stirrup). In some cases of CHL, surgical intervention can help restore hearing function.

What is a processing disorder?

Hearing loss is often defined in terms of the amount of lost volume that results from either a SNHL or a CHL. However, many patients, even those with normal hearing levels, can have a processing disorder that will limit their ability to understand and follow speech in background noise. The noise cancellation feature in NeuroTechnology™ provides significant benefit by reducing background noise and enhancing speech—even for those with normal hearing.

Should I bring a family member with me to my appointment(s)?

I answer this with a decisive ***YES***. Your hearing loss not only impacts you but also everybody around you. I have always encouraged every patient to bring a spouse or a loved one to every appointment so he or she can help me, and the patient, better understand the daily impact of hearing loss on everybody's life.

What is NeuroTechnology™?

In recent years, traditional hearing aids, which simply make sounds louder, have been phased out and replaced with NeuroTechnology™. The significant cognitive benefits to NeuroTechnology™ include: ***binaural processing*** (two ears working together), ***sound orientation*** (ability to detect the source of incoming sounds with increased accuracy), ***enhanced clarity of voices*** (even soft speakers), automatic ***adaptation to environment*** (no more pushing buttons and adjusting volume), and ***noise-cancellation*** filtering of background noise to enhance hearing conversation in noisy environments (hearing better in crowded rooms, restaurants, etc.).

What is the primary benefit of NeuroTechnology™?

This answer is outlined in greater detail throughout the book. In summary, recent reports find that NeuroTechnology™ and the treatment of hearing loss can significantly improve quality of life, reduce the risk of developing dementia, and offer an increase in cognitive function. Yes, all of this can be achieved by treating your hearing loss.

How do I get started with NeuroTechnology™?

It's simple: Request an appointment with the local audiology clinic that sent you this book, or visit ***www.ExcellenceinAudiology.org*** to find a member-clinic in your area. Most clinics will offer a free initial consultation to see if you are a good candidate for hearing loss treatment.

Is getting traditional hearing aids still effective treatment for hearing loss?

For the majority of patients, traditional hearing aids will not effectively treat hearing loss or the symptoms of hearing loss, including tinnitus. Traditional hearing aids are volume-enhancing devices that may help certain people in very limited environments (e.g. conversing one-on-one in a room with ***no*** background noise). For patients needing to follow conversation in dynamic environments (e.g. sitting at a dinner table with family and friends, going out to a restaurant, sitting in a lecture hall or a place of worship, playing cards with others, etc.), NeuroTechnology™ will restore clarity and enhance speech even in background noise.

What are some of my payment options besides insurance?

One way many patients pay for their NeuroTechnology™ is by utilizing Flexible Spending through their work insurance plan, financing at 0% or a fixed rate, or even taking advantage of the new Treatment4Life™ program offered by many of the Excellence in Audiology member-clinics.

What if I need an emergency appointment before or after office hours?

(This answer is a bit longer than most because of the seriousness of some audiology emergencies)

Audiology emergencies most often fall in to one of two categories:

Sudden change in hearing

While rare, a sudden change in hearing can occur. This medical condition, known as *sudden-onset sensorineural hearing loss*, may occur in one, or both (even more rare), ears and is often associated with a virus (and sometimes occurs in tandem with an upper respiratory infection)

There is varying data on successful treatment protocols for this disorder; regardless, the key to potentially recovering hearing function requires seeking medical attention within 24–48 hours of initial symptoms.

Emergency related to the NeuroTechnology™

Broken or "non-functioning devices" may occur from time to time during your treatment. If there is any disturbance, such as lost domes, tight speaker wires, or irritation, call your hearing care provider's office as soon as possible to have them evaluate the urgency of the problem and schedule you to be seen accordingly. In the interim, here are helpful hints to remedy some of the problems that you may encounter until you can be seen in the office:

- If a device is itching your ear, use some ear lotion included in your treatment package.
- A device causing feedback or "squealing" can generally be worn until you are seen by our team. Call the office as soon as you notice this feedback or squealing so that we can schedule you to make a prescription change.

- A dome, earmold, or removable device that is not fitting well, is not to be worn until it can be properly adjusted at the office. Call the office as soon as possible to have your specialists make the adjustment for comfort and fit.

If you are experiencing an audiology emergency that can't wait for regular office hours, most audiology offices have a special number to call either before or after business hours. If you can wait until the office is open, most offices will have special emergency appointments set aside each day to help in these situations.

Can NeuroTechnology™ get wet?

Unlike traditional hearing aids that had no moisture resistance, most of today's NeuroTechnology™ comes with an IP57 rating for dust and moisture resistance. In lay terms, the "IP" stands for International Protection Rating and the "5" indicates the unit is Dust Protected (highest score is a 6 on this scale) and the "7" indicates the unit can be immersed in up to one meter of water (that is over three feet!). With that said—we continue to direct patients to not swim or bathe with their NeuroTechnology™.

Should I sleep with my NeuroTechnology™?

It is recommended to not sleep with your NeuroTechnology™ for three reasons:

1. Give your ear a rest—sleeping with the unit can cause discomfort to the pinna and side of the head.
2. It is easier for the unit to fall out when tossing and turning in bed and may get lost
3. It will wear out the batteries in half the time of their intended lifespan if used 24 hours per day.

However, I do have patients that sleep with their NeuroTechnology™ for safety and personal reasons.

How do I regularly clean my NeuroTechnology™?

Like with cleaning your home…clean it a little each day and it won't become such a mess! Your specialist will help you understand daily and monthly routines for maintaining your NeuroTechnology™ at home. Use a lint free cloth and brush (typically provided at your first treatment appointment) to wipe down the unit every day. This will help prevent oils from the skin, dandruff, earwax, and other environmental dust from clogging the microphones and speaker over time. I also encourage my patients to change the "parts" once a month. This includes wax filters (designed to prevent earwax from entering the unit), domes (designed to securely hold the unit in the ear) and microphone filters (included on some NeuroTechnology™ options).

BIBLIOGRAPHY

THE SCIENCE BEHIND EVERYTHING YOU READ IN THIS BOOK

THIS BOOK IS THE RESULT OF OVER 30 YEARS IN HEARING HEALTH CARE. In this time, we have amassed information from our research, through reading scientific publications, in the classroom (as student and teacher), and from directly interacting with patients and their loved ones. Below is a list of references that helped us put together this book and present the information to you in a succinct manner. You can access these manuscripts on Google Scholar and/or Pubmed.

"Active Ageing: A Policy Framework." *The Aging Male* 5, no. 1 (2002), 1-37.

Adult Cognition and Hearing Aids. U of Canterbury. Communication Disorders, 2015.

Agmon, Maayan, Limor Lavie, and Michail Doumas. "The Association between Hearing Loss, Postural Control, and Mobility in Older Adults: A Systematic Review." *Journal of the American Academy of Audiology* 28, no. 6 (2017), 575-588.

"Association of Hearing Impairment and Subsequent Driving Mobility in Older Adults." *The Gerontologist* 55, no. Suppl_2 (2015), 137-138.

Bainbridge, Kathleen E., Howard J. Hoffman, and Catherine C. Cowie. "Diabetes and Hearing Impairment in the United States: Audiometric Evidence from the National Health and Nutrition Examination Survey, 1999 to 2004." *Annals of Internal Medicine* 149, no. 1 (2008), 1.

Bassuk, Shari S., Thomas A. Glass, and Lisa F. Berkman. "Social Disengagement and Incident Cognitive Decline in Community-Dwelling Elderly Persons." *Annals of Internal Medicine* 131, no. 3 (1999), 165.

Bernabei, Roberto, Ubaldo Bonuccelli, Stefania Maggi, Alessandra Marengoni, Alessandro Martini, Maurizio Memo, Sergio Pecorelli, Andrea P. Peracino, Nicola Quaranta, and Roberto Stella. "Hearing loss and cognitive decline in older adults: questions and answers." *Aging Clinical and Experimental Research* 26, no. 6 (2014), 567-573.

Burns, Elizabeth R., Judy A. Stevens, and Robin Lee. "The direct costs of fatal and non-fatal falls among older adults — United States." *Journal of Safety Research* 58 (2016), 99-103.

Cardin, Velia. "Effects of Aging and Adult-Onset Hearing Loss on Cortical Auditory Regions." *Frontiers in Neuroscience* 10 (2016).

Cass, SP. "Alzheimer's Disease and Exercise: A Literature Review." *Curr. Sports Med. Rep*, February 16, 2017.

Chen, David S., Dane J. Genther, Joshua Betz, and Frank R. Lin. "Association Between Hearing Impairment and Self-Reported Difficulty in Physical Functioning." *Journal of the American Geriatrics Society* 62, no. 5 (2014), 850-856.

Chia, Ee-Munn, Jie J. Wang, Elena Rochtchina, Robert R. Cumming, Philip Newall, and Paul Mitchell. "Hearing Impairment and Health-Related Quality of Life: The Blue Mountains Hearing Study." *Ear and Hearing* 28, no. 2 (2007), 187-195.

Collins, John G. "Prevalence of Selected Chronic Conditions: United States, 1983-85." *PsycEXTRA Dataset* (n.d.).

Davidson, JGS. "Older Adults With a Combination of Vision and Hearing Impairment Experience Higher Rates of Cognitive Impairment, Functional Dependence, and Worse Outcomes Across a Set of Quality Indicators." Last modified August 1, 2017.

De Leon, M. J., S. DeSanti, R. Zinkowski, P. D. Mehta, D. Pratico, S. Segal, C. Clark, D. Kerkman, J. DeBernardis, and J. Li. "MRI and CSF studies in the early diagnosis of Alzheimer's disease." *Journal of Internal Medicine* 256, no. 3 (2004), 205-223.

Deal, Jennifer A., Josh Betz, Kristine Yaffe, Tamara Harris, Elizabeth Purchase-Helzner, Suzanne Satterfield, Sheila Pratt, Nandini Govil, Eleanor M. Simonsick, and Frank R. Lin. "Hearing Impairment and Incident Dementia and Cognitive Decline in Older Adults: The Health ABC Study." *The Journals of Gerontology Series A: Biological Sciences and Medical Sciences*, 2016, glw069.

"Dementia Prevention, Intervention, and Care." *Lancet*, July 19, 2017.

Desjardins, Jamie L. "Analysis of Performance on Cognitive Test Measures Before, During, and After 6 Months of Hearing Aid Use: A Single-Subject Experimental Design." *American Journal of Audiology* 25, no. 2 (2016), 127.

Ferreira, Lidiane M., Alberto N. Ramos, and Eveline P. Mendes. "Characterization of tinnitus in the elderly and its possible related disorders." *Brazilian Journal of Otorhinolaryngology*75, no. 2 (2009), 249-255.

Genther, Dane J., Joshua Betz, Sheila Pratt, Kathryn R. Martin, Tamara B. Harris, Suzanne Satterfield, Douglas C. Bauer, Anne B. Newman, Eleanor M. Simonsick, and Frank R. Lin. "Association Between Hearing Impairment and Risk of Hospitalization in Older Adults." *Journal of the American Geriatrics Society* 63, no. 6 (2015), 1146-1152.

Gibrin, PC, AN Ramos Junior, and EP Mendes. "Prevalence of Tinnitus Complaints and Probable Association with Hearing Loss, Diabetes Mellitus and Hypertension in Elderly." *Codas*, 2013.

Gispen, Fiona E., David S. Chen, Dane J. Genther, and Frank R. Lin. "Association Between Hearing Impairment and Lower Levels of Physical Activity in Older Adults." *Journal of the American Geriatrics Society* 62, no. 8 (2014), 1427-1433.

Govender, SM, CD Govender, and G. Matthews. "Cochlear Function in Patients with Chronic Kidney Disease." *South African/Commun Diord*, December 2013.

Haan, Mary N. "Can Social Engagement Prevent Cognitive Decline in Old Age?" *Annals of Internal Medicine* 131, no. 3 (1999), 220.

"Hearing Impairment and Frailty in English Community-Dwelling Older Adults: A 4-Year Follow-Up Study." *The Gerontologist* 56, no. Suppl_3 (2016), 319-319.

"Hearing Loss and Cognitive Decline in Older Adults." *JAMA Internal Medicine*, February 25, 2013.

"The Impact of Hearing Loss on Quality of Life in Older Adults." *Gerontologist*, October 2003.

"The Impact of Hearing Loss on quality of Life in Older Adults." *Gerontologist*, October 2003.

"An Introduction to MarkeTrak IX: A New Baseline for the Hearing Aid Market." *Hearing Review*, May 15, 2015.

Jacoby, R., and R. Levy. "CT Scanning and the Investigation of Dementia: A Review." *J.R. Soc. Med*, May 1980.

Jamaldeen, Jishana, Aneesh Basheer, Akhil Sarma, and Ravichandran Kandasamy. "Prevalence and patterns of hearing loss among chronic kidney disease patients undergoing haemodialysis." *australasian medical journal*, 2015, 41-46.

Kamil, Rebecca J., Lingsheng Li, and Frank R. Lin. "Association between Hearing Impairment and Frailty in Older Adults." *Journal of the American Geriatrics Society* 62, no. 6 (2014), 1186-1188.

Kelley, Amy S., Kathleen McGarry, Rebecca Gorges, and Jonathan S. Skinner. "The Burden of Health Care Costs for Patients With Dementia in the Last 5 Years of Life." *Annals of Internal Medicine* 163, no. 10 (2015), 729.

Kochkin, Sergei. "MarkeTrak VII." *The Hearing Journal* 60, no. 4 (2007), 24-51.

Lambert, Justin, Rouzbeh Ghadry-Tavi, Kate Knuff, Marc Jutras, Jodi Siever, Paul Mick, Carolyn Roque, Gareth Jones, Jonathan Little, and Harry Miller. "Targeting functional fitness, hearing and health-related quality of life in older adults with hearing loss: Walk, Talk 'n' Listen, study protocol for a pilot randomized controlled trial." *Trials* 18, no. 1 (2017).

Le Goff, Nicolas, Dorothea Wendt, Thomas Lunner, and Elaine Ng. "Opn Clinical Evidence. Oticon White Paper." 2016.

Lin, F.R., L. Ferrucci, Y. An, J.O. Goh, Jimit Doshi, E.J. Metter, C. Davatzikos, M.A. Kraut, and S.M. Resnick. "Association of hearing impairment with brain volume changes in older adults." *NeuroImage* 90 (2014), 84-92.

Lin, Frank R. "Hearing Loss Prevalence in the United States." *Archives of Internal Medicine*171, no. 20 (2011), 1851.

Lin, Frank R. "Hearing Loss and Falls Among Older Adults in the United States." *Archives of Internal Medicine* 172, no. 4 (2012), 369.

Lin, Frank R., E. J. Metter, Richard J. O'Brien, Susan M. Resnick, Alan B. Zonderman, and Luigi Ferrucci. "Hearing Loss and Incident Dementia." *Archives of Neurology* 68, no. 2 (2011).

Martini, Alessandro, Alessandro Castiglione, Roberto Bovo, Antonino Vallesi, and Carlo Gabelli. "Aging, Cognitive Load, Dementia and Hearing Loss." *Audiology and Neurotology* 19, no. 1 (2014), 2-5.

Meister, Hartmut, Stefan Schreitmüller, Magdalene Ortmann, Sebastian Rählmann, and Martin Walger. "Effects of Hearing Loss and Cognitive Load on Speech Recognition with Competing Talkers." *Frontiers in Psychology* 7 (2016).

Melse-Boonstra, Alida, and Ian Mackenzie. "Iodine deficiency, thyroid function and hearing deficit: a review." *Nutrition Research Reviews* 26, no. 02 (2013), 110-117.

Meyerhoff, William L. "The Thyroid and Audition." *The Laryngoscope* 86, no. 4 (1976), 483-489.

Miyawaki, Christina E., E. D. Bouldin, G. S. Kumar, and L. C. McGuire. "Associations between physical activity and cognitive functioning among middle-aged and older adults." *The journal of nutrition, health & aging* 21, no. 6 (2016), 637-647.

Mulrow, Cynthia D., Christine Aguilar, James E. Endicott, Ramon Velez, Michael R. Tuley, Walter S. Charlip, and Judith A. Hill. "Association Between Hearing Impairment and the Quality of Life of Elderly Individuals." *Journal of the American Geriatrics Society* 38, no. 1 (1990), 45-50.

Oh, Esther, Frank Lin, and Sara Mamo. "Enhancing Communication in Adults with Dementia and Age-Related Hearing Loss." *Seminars in Hearing* 38, no. 02 (2017), 177-183.

Palmer, Andrew D., Jason T. Newsom, and Karen S. Rook. "How does difficulty communicating affect the social relationships of older adults? An exploration using data from a national survey." *Journal of Communication Disorders* 62 (2016), 131-146.

Popelka, Michael M., Karen J. Cruickshanks, Terry L. Wiley, Theodore S. Tweed, Barbara E. Klein, and Ronald Klein. "Low Prevalence of Hearing Aid Use Among Older Adults with Hearing Loss: The Epidemiology of Hearing Loss Study." *Journal of the American Geriatrics Society* 46, no. 9 (1998), 1075-1078.

Qian, Z. J., Peter D. Chang, Gul Moonis, and Anil K. Lalwani. "A novel method of quantifying brain atrophy associated with age-related hearing loss." *NeuroImage: Clinical* 16 (2017), 205-209.

Qian, Zhen J., Kapil Wattamwar, Francesco F. Caruana, Jenna Otter, Matthew J. Leskowitz, Barbara Siedlecki, Jaclyn B. Spitzer, and Anil K. Lalwani. "Hearing Aid Use is Associated with Better Mini-Mental State Exam Performance." *The American Journal of Geriatric Psychiatry* 24, no. 9 (2016), 694-702.

Ryu, Nam-Gyu, Il J. Moon, Hayoung Byun, Sun H. Jin, Heesung Park, Kyu-Sun Jang, and Yang-Sun Cho. "Clinical effectiveness of wireless CROS (contralateral routing of offside signals) hearing aids." *European Archives of Oto-Rhino-Laryngology* 272, no. 9 (2014), 2213-2219.

Seimetz, Bruna, Adriane Teixeira, Leticia Rosito, Leticia Flores, Carlos Pappen, and Celso Dall'igna. "Pitch and Loudness Tinnitus in Individuals with Presbycusis." *International Archives of Otorhinolaryngology* 20, no. 04 (2016), 321-326.

Sindhusake, Doungkamol, Paul Mitchell, Philip Newall, Maryanne Golding, Elena Rochtchina, and George Rubin. "Prevalence and characteristics of tinnitus in older adults: the Blue Mountains Hearing Study: Prevalencia y características del acúfeno en adultos mayores: el Estudio de Audición Blue Mountains." *International Journal of Audiology* 42, no. 5 (2003), 289-294.

Snapp, Hillary A., Fred D. Holt, Xuezhong Liu, and Suhrud M. Rajguru. "Comparison of Speech-in-Noise and Localization Benefits in Unilateral Hearing Loss Subjects Using Contralateral Routing of Signal Hearing Aids or Bone-Anchored Implants." *Otology & Neurotology* 38, no. 1 (2017), 11-18.

"Social Isolation in Community-Dwelling Seniors: An Evidence-Based Analysis." *Health Quality Ontario*, August 2008.

Spulber, Gabriela, Eini Niskanen, Stuart MacDonald, Oded Smilovici, Kewei Chen, Eric M. Reiman, Anne M. Jauhiainen, Merja Hallikainen, Susanna Tervo, and Lars-Olof Wahlund. "Whole brain atrophy rate predicts progression from MCI to Alzheimer's disease." *Neurobiology of Aging* 31, no. 9 (2010), 1601-1605.

Su, Peijen, Chih-Chao Hsu, Hung-Ching Lin, Wei-Shin Huang, Tsung-Lin Yang, Wei-Ting Hsu, Cheng-Li Lin, Chung-Yi Hsu, Kuang-Hsi Chang, and Yi-Chao Hsu. "Age-related hearing loss and dementia: a 10-year national population-based study." *European Archives of Oto-Rhino-Laryngology* 274, no. 5 (2017), 2327-2334.

Vignesh, S. S., V. Jaya, Anand Moses, and A. Muraleedharan. "Identifying Early Onset of Hearing Loss in Young Adults With Diabetes Mellitus Type 2 Using High Frequency Audiometry." *Indian Journal of Otolaryngology and Head & Neck Surgery* 67, no. 3 (2014), 234-237.

Weinstein, Barbara E. *Hearing Impairment and Social Isolation in the Elderly*. publisher not identified, 1980.

Yates, J.A., L. Clare, and B. Woods. "You've Got a Friend in Me: Can Social Engagement Mediate the Relationship Between Mood and MCI?" *Innovation in Aging* 1, no. suppl_1 (2017), 1179-1179.

Yates, Jennifer A., Linda Clare, and Robert T. Woods. "What is the Relationship between Health, Mood, and Mild Cognitive Impairment?" *Journal of Alzheimer's Disease* 55, no. 3 (2016), 1183-1193.

Zheng, Yuqiu, Shengnuo Fan, Wang Liao, Wenli Fang, Songhua Xiao, and Jun Liu. "Hearing impairment and risk of Alzheimer's disease: a meta-analysis of prospective cohort studies." *Neurological Sciences* 38, no. 2 (2016), 233-239.

IF YOU READ THIS BOOK, chances are that you or a family member are struggling to deal with impact of hearing loss on your social, physical, and mental well-being. By now, we hope you have come to understand the negative impact of untreated hearing loss on overall quality of life and cognitive function.

We thank you for taking your hearing healthcare seriously and for allowing us to provide the education necessary for you to make an informed decision about medically treating your hearing loss.

When you are ready to take the next step to improve your life, your cognitive function, and your hearing health, please call:

(310) 421-4396

to Schedule Your Treatment

South Bay Hearing